Musculoskeletal Pain – Assessment, Prediction and Treatment

A pragmatic approach

T0187094

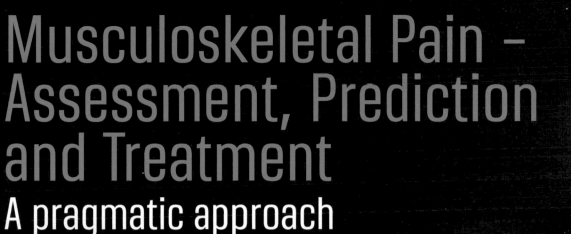

Musculoskeletal Pain – Assessment, Prediction and Treatment

A pragmatic approach

David M Walton

James M Elliott

Forewords Guy Simoneau

Wellington K. Hsu

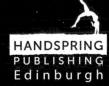

HANDSPRING
PUBLISHING
Edinburgh

HANDSPRING PUBLISHING LIMITED
The Old Manse, Fountainhall,
Pencaitland, East Lothian
EH34 5EY, Scotland
Tel: +44 1875 341 859
Website: www.handspringpublishing.com

First published 2020 in the United Kingdom by Handspring Publishing
Copyright © Handspring Publishing 2020

ISBN 978-1-912085-50-7
ISBN (Kindle eBook) 97-1 -912085-51-4

British Library Cataloguing in Publication Data
A catalogue record for this book is available from the British Library

Library of Congress Cataloguing in Publication Data
A catalog record for this book is available from the Library of Congress

Notice
Neither the Publisher nor the Authors assume any responsibility for any loss or injury and/or damage to persons or property arising out of or relating to any use of the material contained in this book. It is the responsibility of the treating practitioner, relying on independent expertise and knowledge of the patient, to determine the best treatment and method of application for the patient.

All reasonable efforts have been made to obtain copyright clearance for illustrations in the book for which the authors or publishers do not own the rights. If you believe that one of your illustrations has been used without such clearance please contact the publishers and we will ensure that appropriate credit is given in the next reprint.

Commissioning Editor Mary Law
Project Manager Morven Dean
Copy Editor Susan Stuart
Designer Bruce Hogarth
Indexer Aptara, India
Typesetter DSM Soft, India
Printer Melita, Malta

The
Publisher's
policy is to use
paper manufactured
from sustainable forests

CONTENTS

DEDICATION

This book is dedicated to the wonderful women in our lives – they have made us better sons, husbands, fathers, thinkers, researchers, teachers, and collaborators.

My mother Marilyn, my wife Amanda, my daughters Hannah and Ashlyn, and my mentors Bev Padfield, Dr. Jayne Garland and Dr. Joy MacDermid.

David M. Walton

My mother Nancy, my wife Helen, my daughters Emma and Zoë, and my mentor and friend, Emeritus Professor, Gwen Jull.

James M. Elliott

Dave Walton BScPT, MSc, PhD (@uwo_dwalton)

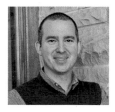

Dave completed his Bachelor of Science in Physical Therapy in 1999 from Western University in London Ontario, Canada. He worked as a clinician from 1999 to 2010 while also completing a Master's degree in neuroscience and a PhD in Health and Rehabilitation Sciences from Western. He is currently an Associate Professor with the School of Physical Therapy at Western University with a cross-appointment to the Dept. of Psychiatry in Western's Schulich School of Medicine and Dentistry, and he holds an Honorary Associate Professor title with the Discipline of Physiotherapy at the University of Sydney (NSW, Australia). He is Director and Lead Researcher of the Pain and Quality of Life Integrative Research Lab (www.pirlresearch.com) at which he leads a team of 16 graduate students, volunteers, honours students and high school co-op students. He also holds the positions of Associate Scientist with the Lawson Health Research Institute, Associate Scientist with Western's Bone and Joint Institute, and is an Associate Editor for the scientific journal *Musculoskeletal Science and Practice*.

Dave has been recognized by his peers for exceptional contributions to research, teaching, mentorship, and service to the profession of physiotherapy. He has twice been awarded the Faculty of Health Sciences Teaching Excellence Award and has been nominated for Western's highest teaching awards including the Marilyn Robinson Teaching Award of Excellence and the Provost's Award for Collaborative Teaching. He has been awarded Early Career Researcher awards through the Canadian Pain Society and the Ontario Ministry of Research and Innovation, and was the 2014 recipient of the National Mentorship Award through the Canadian Physiotherapy Association. In 2016 he became the first person in Western University's history to hold the titles of Teaching Fellow and Faculty Scholar simultaneously. In 2018 he became the first physiotherapist to be named a Mayday Pain and Society Fellow, that same year he was a member of the Steering Committee for the Global Year for Excellence in Pain Education through the International Association for the Study of Pain. He was co-founder and Chair of the Canadian Physiotherapy Association's Pain Science Division and is the developer and Field Leader of Canada's first competency-based Master's level degree program in Interprofessional Pain Management.

Dave's current research work focuses on measurement of pain and related experiences, including both psychometrics and critical measurement theory, as well as understanding mechanisms of the acute to recovery/chronic pain cascade through integrative biological, psychological, and social analyses. In 2017 he travelled across Canada to better understand the current state of physiotherapy and its future directions during the Physio Moves Canada project, and he is now engaged in research and practice in educational and training reform and innovation for pre- and post-professional development. He has produced over 100 scientific peer-reviewed publications and has presented his work globally at national and international professional events and conferences. He has been invited to speak at several recent events regarding the future of physiotherapy and rehabilitation in Canada.

On a personal level, Dave can most commonly be found hanging out with his wife, two daughters, and dog, most likely in front of a barbecue or eating a butter tart (a unique Canadian treat). He holds black belts in Tae Kwon Do and Aikido, and despite the years he still enjoys a bit of breakdancing and salsa dancing from time to time. He is a fan of American football, the blues harmonica, and the Toronto Blue Jays baseball club.

James 'Jim' Elliott, PT, PhD (@ElliottJSyd)

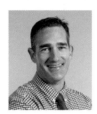

Jim completed his PhD at the University of Queensland, Australia (UQ) in 2007 and a post-doctoral fellowship (2010) at UQ's CCRE-Spine. The primary focus of his interdisciplinary laboratory is to quantify altered spinal cord anatomy and whole-body skeletal muscle degeneration as potential markers of recovery following spinal trauma. His work has resulted in external recognition as a global expert in neck pain (broadly) and whiplash injuries (more specifically).

He is currently a Professor of Allied Health in the Faculty of Health Sciences at the University of Sydney and the Northern Sydney Local Health District at the Kolling Research Institute. Prior to this, Jim was a tenure-track Associate Professor in the Feinberg School of Medicine at Northwestern University in Chicago, USA, where he remains an adjunct Professor and principal investigator of the Neuromuscular Imaging Research Laboratory.

He currently serves as an Advisory Board Member for the journal *Spine* and is an advisory member to the Board of Directors for the *Journal of Orthopaedic & Sports Physical Therapy*. Jim was the recipient of the 2011 Eugene Michels New Investigator Award from the American Physical Therapy Association, the 2015 Faculty Award for Engagement from Northwestern's Graduate School, and the 2017 Ver Steeg Faculty Award for Excellence in work with graduate students. He was recognised as a Catherine Worthingham Fellow of the American Physical Therapy Association in 2018.

On a personal note, Jim played professional baseball for the San Diego Padres (1990-1992), worked in major league baseball operations for the Colorado Rockies (1993-1996) and was inducted into the University of Denver Athletic Hall of Fame (2014). He thoroughly enjoys banging on his drum set, spending time with his wife and three children, and admits to needing medication for his life-long love of the Chicago Cubs.

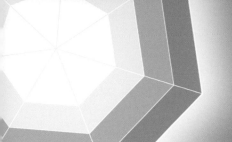

This book presents a common-sense approach to interpreting and applying existing clinical knowledge and new research to help clinicians make sense of the complex phenomena of acute and chronic post-traumatic musculoskeletal pain. Built upon the *Assess, Predict, Treat* framework, the book offers a method to help clinicians better understand their patients' pain, presents evidence-based decision tools to predict natural and clinical course of common conditions such as neck and low back pain, and then synthesizes that information into a logical integrated treatment approach that respects the individuality of the patient, the experiences of the clinician, and the value of evidence-informed practice. Written by two global leaders in the field of post-traumatic pain and recovery, the book provides a valuable framework to facilitate novice clinicians in their transition to becoming clinical experts, and helps mid- and late-stage clinicians better interpret, synthesize, and discuss complex information on pain with the goal of optimized outcomes on a patient-by-patient basis.

How did we get here?

It all started inside an MRI tube in Brisbane, Australia. Jim Elliott, in the middle of a post-doctoral fellowship at the University of Queensland, was conducting a study exploring the hypothesis that some component of the experience of neck pain is explainable by the quality and composition of the neck muscles, with a specific focus on fatty infiltration in the space between muscle cells. He had developed this hypothesis while working as a clinician in Denver, Colorado where he spent much of his days evaluating and providing treatment recommendations for people with chronic neck pain. Many of these people could trace the genesis of their pain back to a traumatic event, commonly a motor vehicle crash that resulted in a diagnosis of *whiplash associated disorder*, as it had been recently defined.

After a shoulder injury ended his professional baseball career, Jim had graduated from the (then) Masters of Science in Physical Therapy (MSPT) program at Regis University in Denver. Working in Denver he consistently saw what he *thought* were poor quality neck muscles in several of his patients. As so often happens, a clinical observation leads to a number of research questions, and Jim started knocking on doors of other medical and rehab experts to ask if they too had identified this clinical finding. Most provided the standard take on the issue at the time, that those with chronic neck pain, especially when arising from the highly litigious context of motor vehicle injury, were most likely too fearful of pain or just lazy, and as a result were demonstrating muscle atrophy and fatty infiltration. Some even offered the suggestion that these people must have been obese, hence the increased intramuscular fat. Jim found this wholly unsatisfactory – he was practicing in Colorado, a state full of health-conscious, outdoorsy-type people. The old disuse and obese explanations just did not sit well.

After six years of clinical practice, and five years of combined PhD and clinical work, Jim defended his PhD thesis in 2007 that focused on the composition of neck muscles following whiplash injuries from a motor vehicle collision. Feeling the work was not yet complete, he immediately jumped at the opportunity to pursue a post-doctoral fellowship that would last for three years at the University of Queensland in Brisbane. So, he and his lovely wife Helen, packed up with two young girls and a son on the way, and moved the whole clan to the other side of the world.

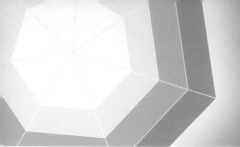

Mcanwhile Dave Walton, a graduate of the (then) Bachelor of Science program in Physical Therapy from the University of Western Ontario, was contemplating his own transition from clinician to academic. After completing a neuroscience-focused Master of Science degree he had stepped away from academia and began working as a clinical physiotherapist in southwestern Ontario, Canada. Like so many other young physios, he assumed that sports rehab was his calling. He pursued many of the classic routes of continuing professional development for those on that path, though after focusing almost exclusively on manual therapy training for five years he was unsatisfied by his inability to really understand his patients with complex and chronic problems.

It was about this time, in the first half of the 2000s, that a movement was quietly growing in the PT world that was challenging the way providers viewed the phenomenon of pain. Ground zero for much of this work seemed to be Australia, where researchers were using visual illusions and targeted educational strategies to understand and treat pain that appealed to Dave's interests in neuroscience and cognitions. A voracious appetite for everything pain-related ensued, and by 2006 he was ready to return to academia to pursue a PhD with a focus on non-medical chronic pain management. While he entered his PhD training with a plan to create the newest, hottest, chronic pain intervention, it became quickly apparent that there was no consensus on what *caused* some people to develop chronic pain after injury. Prescribing to a belief that it's hard to treat something when you don't know what caused it, a slight pivot led him toward the fields of psychology, pain measurement and prognosis with a focus on WAD as the study model. Four years later he

defended his thesis describing the development of a new 'chronic pain risk screening tool' (that would eventually become the Traumatic Injuries Distress Scale) in 2010. Serendipity intervened and he was offered a tenure-track faculty position right out of his PhD work. But recognizing that all 10 years of training and three degrees had been completed at the same institution, he negotiated time and resources for a self-funded mini post-doctoral experience in Australia, with most of that time to be spent at the University of Queensland.

And this brings us to the MRI tube. Having heard about Jim's work being conducted out of the imaging suite of one of the major hospitals in Brisbane, Dave was keen to see it in action. One afternoon in late July 2010 he made his way to the hospital with the intention of observing the MRI-based data collection. Within an hour of arrival Dave was in nothing more than his underwear and a hospital gown, preparing to enter the tube as one of Jim's 'healthy control' study participants. These were still early days in Jim's research program, and with his consent Dave was invited to spend a little extra time in the tube so they could trial different image acquisition parameters. Two hours later two things had happened: 1) Dave learned he had mild claustrophobia; and 2) a new friendship had emerged that would become a strong and ongoing collaborative relationship. Dave returned to Western to start his full-time academic career in September, and Jim finished his post-doc work and was back in his home town of Chicago to begin his own tenure-track position at Northwestern University later that same year.

Both being collaborative by nature, the two realized early that they would both be more successful

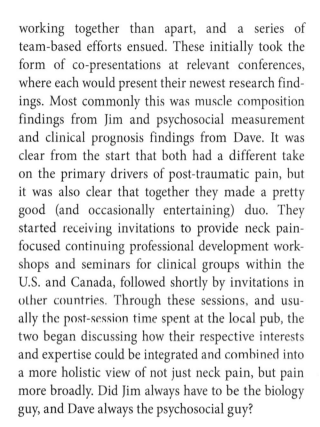

working together than apart, and a series of team-based efforts ensued. These initially took the form of co-presentations at relevant conferences, where each would present their newest research findings. Most commonly this was muscle composition findings from Jim and psychosocial measurement and clinical prognosis findings from Dave. It was clear from the start that both had a different take on the primary drivers of post-traumatic pain, but it was also clear that together they made a pretty good (and occasionally entertaining) duo. They started receiving invitations to provide neck pain-focused continuing professional development workshops and seminars for clinical groups within the U.S. and Canada, followed shortly by invitations in other countries. Through these sessions, and usually the post-session time spent at the local pub, the two began discussing how their respective interests and expertise could be integrated and combined into a more holistic view of not just neck pain, but pain more broadly. Did Jim always have to be the biology guy, and Dave always the psychosocial guy?

By this time the field, that had become broadly defined by the colloquial term 'pain science', had evolved to the point that most people accepted pain could not be easily reduced to a single mechanism, whether biological, psychological, or social. The two began sketching out the idea of a multidomain understanding of musculoskeletal pain, representing a move away from the popular approach of mechanistically distinct 'subgrouping', towards more holistic phenotyping wherein *multiple drivers* could exist in the same person with each contributing relatively more or less to the patient's pain experience. Hence the concept of the radar plot was born, and through continued discussions,

the importance of triangulating findings through diverse sources of knowledge fitted with their own understandings of musculoskeletal pain, prognosis and treatment.

In true academic style, they started working to complicate the framework before even setting it free in the wild. There are currently versions of the radar plot with more points, different descriptors, and arrows indicating likely interactional relationships between the different domains. Yet it became clear very quickly that what clinicians wanted was something better and more informative than what they had become so used to, that was also easily understandable and a useful communicative tool. Hence the domains, their complex interactions, and multivariate contributions to pain were scaled back to the seven domains presented in this book. And in hindsight, this was the right decision.

Today, Jim and Dave have continued their own evolution as research academics, adopting new epistemic frameworks and broadening their focus to the larger field of trauma and pain more generally, but they continue to dedicate time to helping clinicians make sense of some very messy topics. After red flags have been cleared, the current iteration of the radar plot appears to capture the majority of drivers of the pain experience that rehabilitation professionals see in their routine clinical practices. It is not perfect, and the entire concept arguably remains too reductionistic to *really* grasp the complexities of the pain experience. But to be honest, no one has *really* grasped these complexities, so presented herein is what is most easily defensible based on the current state of evidence and practice. We believe it is better than what has been available previously, and even today there are few frameworks that seem to be resonating with clinicians in the same way as the radar plot and tri-angulation concepts.

There seems to be something compelling in its simplicity, which as readers of this book will learn, is the end depiction of a complex set of mechanisms and evaluative processes. The points of the plot may well change in future iterations, and the promise of big data-based machine learning algorithms will likely drive this evolution forward even more. For now, and as long as clinicians and their patients continue to value intuition, wisdom, creativity, critical thinking and applicability, we believe the concept of a multi-dimensional framework such as the *Assess, Predict, Treat* approach described in this book will be effective in improving shared clinical decision-making and optimizing pain-related patient outcomes.

David M. Walton, PT, PhD, FCAMPT
Associate Professor, School of Physical Therapy,
Western University, London, ON, Canada
October, 2019

James M. Elliott, PT, PhD, FAPTA
Professor, Northern Sydney Local Health District
and Faculty of Health Sciences,
The University of Sydney, NSW, Australia
Adjunct Professor, NU-PTHMS,
Feinberg School of Medicine,
Northwestern University, Chicago, IL, USA
October, 2019

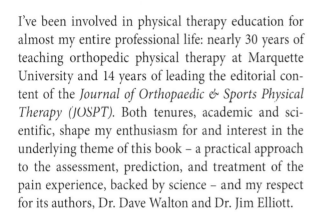

I've been involved in physical therapy education for almost my entire professional life: nearly 30 years of teaching orthopedic physical therapy at Marquette University and 14 years of leading the editorial content of the *Journal of Orthopaedic & Sports Physical Therapy (JOSPT)*. Both tenures, academic and scientific, shape my enthusiasm for and interest in the underlying theme of this book – a practical approach to the assessment, prediction, and treatment of the pain experience, backed by science – and my respect for its authors, Dr. Dave Walton and Dr. Jim Elliott.

In the scientific arena, I've worked directly with Drs. Walton and Elliott on many occasions, most recently on the coordination of two very well-received special issues for *JOSPT* on whiplash associated disorders. I've also made a point over the years to attend their sessions at professional meetings, knowing that Dave and Jim would deliver engaging and effective presentations of their work. As an educator, the first time I heard Dave and Jim present their three-pronged 'Assess, Predict, Treat' framework, I recall being intrigued by the novelty of reframing a model I was already familiar with, specifically the management of musculoskeletal disorders, into a model for the management of musculoskeletal *pain*, which espoused a more comprehensive and prognosis-informed biopsychosocial approach to the assessment and treatment of the pain experience. It fundamentally changed my approach to interpretation of the literature and teaching.

I am excited for the community of clinicians, researchers and educators that *Musculoskeletal Pain – Assessment, Prediction, and Treatment* has arrived on the scene. This book represents the culmination of the authors' extensive clinical experience and clinically

oriented research. Furthermore, the text is written in the same dynamic and engaging style that has garnered both authors recognition as exceptional educators. Dr. Walton, Associate Professor with the School of Physical Therapy at Western University (London, Canada), is the author of more than 100 scientific publications. His research and knowledge translation efforts concentrate on the management of neuromusculoskeletal pain, through a focus on measurement and evaluation, predicting outcomes, and translating new knowledge into practice. He has led or co-led interdisciplinary research groups and initiatives to improve pain research, education, and practice at both national and global levels. Dr. Elliott, Professor at the University of Sydney in Australia and Adjunct Professor at Northwestern University in Chicago, has established himself as one of the premier researchers in the world in the field of cervical spine injuries resulting from motor-vehicle collisions. His work with new imaging technology combined with novel perspectives on the management of whiplash injuries has resulted in the publication of more than 100 scientific journal articles. Both authors are internationally recognized scholars who have focused on conducting research designed to make a positive impact on the provision of clinical care.

In *Musculoskeletal Pain – Assessment, Prediction, and Treatment*, the authors present a pragmatic approach to the management of musculoskeletal pain, describing a comprehensive and yet manageable plan for assessing a person's pain and disability experience, using a seven-point radar plot to create a profile representative of the various components of the biopsychosocial model. A fundamental aspect of the authors' 'Assess, Predict, Treat' framework is making informed decisions on treatment in part based on our current knowledge related to recovery and potential factors that may impact that recovery process either positively or negatively. This is a paradigm shift in the management of people with musculoskeletal pain.

Of special note is the success that Drs. Walton and Elliott achieved in translating 'the complexity of the pain experience' into a clinically relevant framework and, in the process, synthesizing significant advances made over the past decade or so in understanding pain mechanisms and psychosocial features affecting musculoskeletal pain.

The publication of this book, written by these two authors, could not have been a timelier event: a unique resource with true potential for significant positive impact on education and practice as they relate to the management of musculoskeletal pain conditions.

Congratulations to Dave and Jim on this remarkable and meaningful accomplishment!

Guy G. Simoneau, PT, PhD, FAPTA
Editor-in-Chief Emeritus,
Journal of Orthopaedic & Sports Physical Therapy
Professor in Physical Therapy,
Marquette University, Milwaukee, WI, USA
October, 2019

Musculoskeletal pain afflicts millions of individuals worldwide both as acute and chronic, as well as continuous and intermittent problems. As a spine surgeon, I am reminded daily of the dramatic impact of these pain conditions on patients' lives. Based on their societal burden, there are not enough resources available in the world to dedicate to these prevalent and detrimental disease processes. If not dealt with thoughtfully, strategically, and methodically, musculoskeletal pain can destroy relationships, fulfillment, and overall quality of life of the patients we see every day.

Musculoskeletal Pain – Assessment, Prediction and Treatment, authored by the esteemed Drs. David Walton and James Elliott, equips healthcare practitioners with a roadmap and comprehensive toolbox to help improve lives affected by pain. The innovative approach outlined by Walton and Elliott helps organize pain components into separate domains that each require different types of treatment. This strategy, which identifies and introduces quality evidence-based literature when applicable, provides a systematic algorithm for treatment for an entire population of patients with musculoskeletal pain – all of whom are different from each other. In a field where clinical decisions are commonly made with mere anecdotal or experiential opinions, this book changes the paradigm by emphasizing and organizing the available evidence in support of mechanisms of pain coupled with multiple treatment options. This book recognizes that complex pain patients require an inordinate amount of time to properly identify the sources and domains of discomfort to optimize outcomes. Healthcare practitioners are often blinded by their specialized knowledge base which forces the categorization of patients along a similar diagnosis leading to one generic treatment strategy. The lessons of Walton and Elliott highlight the danger of that approach and propose a paradigm shift to help patients in need. It is important to familiarize all healthcare practitioners who treat these patients with the systematic assessments of pain origin.

I cannot think of two more qualified, insightful, and forward-thinking academicians to author this book. Recognizing that at least 90% of chronic pain patients should be treated with conservative care, Drs. Walton and Elliott harbor a philosophical background rooted in rehabilitation that has demonstrated the most promising long-term results in treating these symptoms. Furthermore, Dr. Walton has built a wonderful career in both teaching and research at Western University in London, Ontario. He has dedicated his current research to the investigation of mechanisms of the acute and chronic pain cascade and been recognized as a global thought leader in this field. I admire Dr. Elliott as a close collaborator and colleague and feel fortunate to have worked with him during his productive years as an Associate Professor at Northwestern University. It is not only his analytical mind and progressive mindset that has separated him as an opinion leader, but also his compassion and empathy that are obvious during discussions of these topics that make him perfect for this treatise.

It is my honor to highlight the importance of the pragmatic lessons in this book for all therapists of patients with musculoskeletal pain. After having read the book, I consider myself astronomically better equipped to deal with the needs of the chronic pain patients I treat on a regular basis. I trust that you will recognize its practicality and applicability as well.

Wellington K. Hsu, MD
Clifford C. Raisbeck Distinguished Professor
of Orthopaedic Surgery
Director of Research
Professor, Department of Orthopaedic Surgery
Professor, Department of Neurological Surgery
Northwestern University
Feinberg School of Medicine
Chicago, IL, USA
October, 2019

1

A Pragmatic Approach to Seeing the Invisible

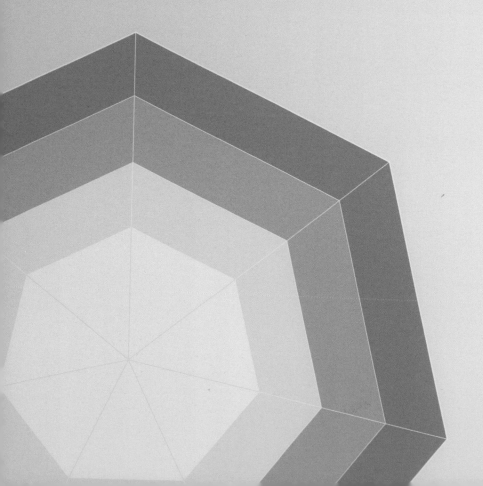

Introduction to this book

This book has been written as an introductory guide to a new framework for thinking about pain and its related sequelae. We have collated several decades' worth of collective work in the fields of pain measurement, mechanisms, and management as clinicians, educators and researchers, to arrive at this framework. The first few chapters will introduce the *Assess, Predict, Treat (APT)* paradigms, including the concepts of the radar plot and triangulation, and provide readers who are new to the field with a bit of a 'crash course' on pain and some of the controversies and ambiguities surrounding it. The second half of this book will delve deeper into each of the primary pain drivers of our radar plot concept. Each of these chapters is structured similarly, starting with a description of the mechanism itself and some background into how each may influence a patient's experience or report of pain. These are followed by suggestions for how to identify each domain as a likely/not likely pain driver (*Assess*), including a table that roughly indicates the shift in certainty that a domain is/is not an important driver for that patient. Then we present current evidence that can be used to predict either the natural course, or the outcomes of treatment in a patient who presents with that domain as a strong driver (*Predict*). Finally, we close each of those chapters with discussion on current evidence, or when that does not exist, recommendations from our own experiences, as ways to improve the experiences of pain for a patient with that domain as a primary driver (*Treat*). Of note, the intervention sections are often the least rich, largely because, despite decades of research, the evidence is simply not strong in a lot of these areas. We would argue that part of the reason for that is that prior researchers have not attempted to recruit patients according to a structured *phenotyping* framework like we are proposing here (i.e. instead all patients are often taken as though they are considered equal). One of our hopes by presenting the APT framework is that researchers and clinicians can use them to make more informed (or 'apt' – get it?) decisions about people in pain, and in doing so will lead to research with greater clinical impact.

With that, we start by exploring the construct of pain and the challenges associated with research and clinical intervention for a largely invisible experience.

Pain as a latent construct

The study of pain has matured into a well-recognized academic discipline over the past century, gaining particular steam over the past 50 years. Hundreds of texts and thousands of peer-reviewed papers on the subject have been published, spanning basic sciences to clinical translation. As a result, and in the interest of providing context for several of the following sections, we need not reiterate what several authors before us have said. Instead, we will summarize the phenomenon of a pain experience in general, and as it pertains to musculoskeletal pain and associated disability on a patient-by-patient basis more specifically. For those interested, some of our favorite and seminal texts, which have shaped our own clinical curiosities and research on the mysterious phenomenon of pain, are listed in Box 1.1.

Box 1.1 Selected additional readings

Butler, D., Moseley, L., 2013. *Explain Pain*, 2nd edition, NOI Group.

Caudill, M., 2016. *Managing Pain Before It Manages You,* 4th edition, The Guilford Press.

Jackson, M., 2003. *Pain: The Science and Culture of Why We Hurt*, Vintage Canada.

Melzack, R., Wall, P.D., 1996. *The Challenge of Pain*, 2nd edition, Penguin Books.

Moseley, L., 2008. *Painful Yarns,* Dancing Giraffe Press.

Turk, D., Melzack, R., 2010. *The Handbook of Pain Assessment,* 3rd edition, The Guilford Press.

To understand pain, and to understand the value of subsequent concepts like triangulation and phenotyping (described in later chapters), we must first appreciate pain as a *latent construct*; it cannot be directly observed. At best the experience of another person's pain can be inferred from different but related variables or phenomena. That is to say, it would be (nearly) impossible for you to know precisely how much pain someone is experiencing by virtue of looking at them, studying their x-ray images, or reading about their past medical history. However, each of those sources of information (asking the patient, looking at diagnostic images, understanding past history) together will give you a *sense* of what the patient *might* be feeling. We will always be trying to make sense of a patient's experience through the lens of our own experiences with pain, life, and diagnostic procedures, meaning there is currently no objective, measurable, gold-standard diagnostic marker or markers of pain any more than there are objective markers of love, happiness, guilt, religious fervor, etc. All of those phenomena may be estimated or inferred based on your knowledge of the person, their personal and cultural beliefs and values, their prior experiences, current behaviors, and broader contextual factors. Such estimations are imperfect at best. Someone slowly swaying back and forth with their eyes closed may indicate a person listening to a favorite song, entranced in a deep meditative state, or experiencing a bout of syncope – same behaviors but very different experiences. Similarly, physiological markers cannot provide concrete infallible evidence of someone's current experience: dilated pupils, elevated heart rate, and rapid breathing could indicate a person in a state of abject fear as easily as it could be a person in the throes of sexual passion.

Even advancing measurement technologies, such as functional magnetic resonance imaging (fMRI, Box 1.2), are an inexact estimation of whether someone is in pain, let alone how much pain they are in. This is true in most cases, though recent research has indicated that by combining fMRI data with computerized machine learning, it may be possible to train an artificial intelligence (AI) to predict the intensity of a person's pain experience if the AI is first fed hundreds of scans of that person's brain activity under 'control'

Box 1.2 Functional magnetic resonance imaging

Functional magnetic resonance imaging (fMRI) is a research tool that uses long-duration serial images of *regional cerebral blood flow* (rCBF) in an awake or sleeping person or animal. The theory posits that brain regions that are neurologically (electrically) active are also more metabolically active and consume more oxygen. As such, the body's circulatory system responds by constricting blood flow to inactive areas so it can shunt additional blood (and hence oxygen) to the active areas. Assuming the person is otherwise perfectly still, changes in fMRI water signal are interpreted as increased cortical perfusion in that region, hence more activity. This is a technique that provides excellent *spatial* resolution (can pinpoint activity to very discrete brain regions), but because changes in circulatory dynamics take some time, offers poor *temporal* resolution (a delay between actual brain activity and the first indication of changed regional perfusion on fMRI). It is a powerful tool when in the right hands and used under very stringent protocols. When protocols are lax however, it may lead researchers to believe that a dead Atlantic salmon is interpreting pictures of human emotions (Bennett et al., 2009).

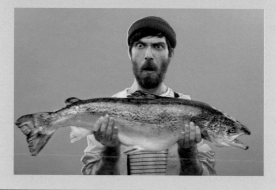

(known pain intensity) conditions. Armed with such a background library of a person's unique *neurosignatures* of pain (activation patterns unique to you), the AI may then become fairly accurate in predicting the *current* experiences by virtue of an existing library of *past* experiences. But without such a rich library of data to draw upon, fMRI or other related neural scanning techniques are imperfect at best, and potentially dangerously inaccurate at worst. Therefore, despite decades of research searching for a concrete, objective and unbiased 'pain-o-meter', we find ourselves forced to continue to accept the eloquent declaration of Margo McCaffery in 1968: "*Pain is whatever the experiencing person says it is, existing whenever the experiencing person says it does*". Despite a lot of hype and a bit of promise, we've yet to find a better solution than that.

All of this poses a challenge to clinicians wanting to benchmark their clinical outcomes in treating patients with pain, in that there is no gold standard against which to compare. The same could be said for other latent constructs such as self-rated disability, distress, fear or anxiety; all of which can go 'hand-in-hand' with reported levels of pain. Such a conundrum also exists for the medicolegal system, that for decades has wrestled with how best to determine the verifiability of a complainant's reports of pain and suffering in the absence of any objective markers. A common legal scenario, either within or beyond the courtroom, is one in which both sets of attorneys nominate their respective medical 'experts' who, after having reviewed hours-to-days' worth of reports and records, each provide their best opinion as to whether it is more (or less) likely than not that the complainant presents with genuine pain. In most cases those opinions differ considerably, leaving a largely uninformed judge or jury to decide whose opinion best supports or refutes the 'but-for' test, which considers whether the plaintiff's complaints or injuries would not have occurred 'but-for' the defendant's negligent act. Often, court decisions and their impacts on people's lives come down to which side's expert the jury likes best.

This also poses several problems for patients who are suffering from what is often considered an *invisible* experience of pain. Pain, especially chronic pain, is somewhat unique as a medical condition in that it is one of the few conditions that leaves sufferers genuinely disappointed when a diagnostic test comes back negative. We've seen this scenario play out countless times in our clinical practices, when a long-suffering patient presents for a visit, clearly dejected that their last set of x-rays or MRI showed 'nothing' to explain their persistent pain. It is plausible such disappointment is largely driven by their interpretation of being the targets of skepticism when describing their pain to clinicians, employers, or even family members. The desire for an observable explanatory sign, something they can point to and say 'See! I told you this wasn't right!' is powerful in most global cultures (Rhodes et al., 1999). This lack of clear structural pathology also appears to cause considerable tension and cognitive dissonance for healthcare providers, many of whom were trained in a biomedical model that prioritized identification of problematic tissues. The experience of chronic pain, and the stigma experienced by those who express it, has been described in several research studies and appears to compound the suffering of those who live in pain and struggle to find legitimacy (Slade et al., 2009; Cohen et al., 2011). Some studies have even found evidence that patients begin to doubt themselves and their ability to distinguish between normal and abnormal states of health after so many experiences with providers who, according to the patient, question or do not believe they are in pain. The public discourse around the opioid crisis that started in earnest near the end of 2016 only added to the problems of people in pain. Not only had they long been the target of skepticism from cynical healthcare providers who saw them as 'complainers', but suddenly they now found themselves labeled as 'drug seekers' or even addicts any time they requested pharmaceutical management for their pain.

The search for concrete objective pain markers has therefore been a priority area of research for years.

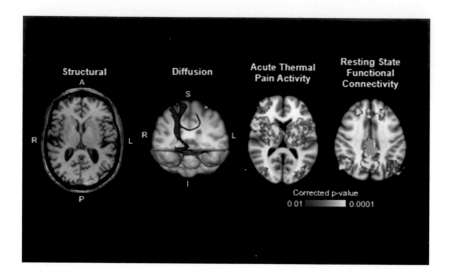

Figure 1.1

Example of structural, diffusion, and functional brain images. The axial structural image was acquired using a 3-D magnetization-prepared rapid gradient-echo, T1-weighted, gradient-echo sequence and can provide morphometric properties of the gray matter. The diffusion example shows a 3-D tractography map using the right ventral posterolateral nucleus of the thalamus as a seed. The axial functional images show average group activation from an acute thermal pain stimulus applied to the lower back, and group average connectivity to the bilateral posterior cingulate cortices (light blue). *A*, Anterior; *I*, inferior; *L*, left; *P*, posterior; *R*, right; *S*, superior. (Reprinted with permission from Crawford, R.J., Fortin, M., Weber, K.A. 2nd, et al., 2019. Are magnetic resonance imaging technologies crucial to our understanding of spinal conditions? *Journal of Orthopaedic & Sports Physical Therapy* 49:320–9. ©Journal of Orthopaedic & Sports Physical Therapy®)

For example, the United States Department of Defense holds a large granting competition each year to fund research specifically focused on identifying biomarkers of pain. Despite some advancements in the field, driven largely by fMRI (Fig. 1.1), genomics, transcriptomics, proteomics and big data analytical techniques, it still seems we are far from accessible, and affordable, objective biomarkers of pain. And the field has yet to reconcile the fact that the search for all such markers continues to be inextricably linked with comparisons against the person's subjective report of pain – that is, the verbal report of pain remains as close to a 'gold standard' as we currently have even with all of the caveats, limitations, and biases inherent in verbal self-report. We do not see how the field will ever reconcile this tension – that despite technology that is exponentially advancing, the study of pain will always rely on what the patient (or research subject) says they are experiencing. Here we lean on the words of Harvard psychologist Daniel Gilbert, author of *Stumbling on Happiness*, when he says:

If we want to know how a person feels, we must begin by acknowledging the fact that there is one and only one observer stationed at the critical point of view. She may not always remember what she felt before, and she may not always be aware of what she is feeling right now. We may be puzzled by her reports, skeptical of her memory, and worried about her ability to use language as we do. But when all our hand wringing is over, we must admit that she is the only person who has even the slightest chance of describing 'the view from in here', which is why her claims serve as the gold standard against which all other measures are measured. (Gilbert, 2006, pp. 72–73)

If we do know anything about pain, it's that the experience and communication thereof is tremendously complex. It has become clear over the past 20 years or so that pain cannot be reduced to a single structural abnormality. A growing collection of research studies has found that abnormalities on diagnostic imaging, from knee pain to shoulder pain to low back or neck pain, are just as common in people without pain as they are in people with pain, raising doubt as to the value of any diagnostic imaging in what are often called 'uncomplicated' cases of pain. Of course, the label of 'uncomplicated' is itself a misnomer – as we're going to see, there is no such thing as a routine and easily understandable pain experience. However, many policy makers in most developed countries have endorsed current guidelines that explicitly recommend *against* use of imaging, and most countries with socialized healthcare systems have delisted such diagnostic procedures meaning that those patients who want an x-ray must pay for it out of pocket. As we will discuss in a subsequent chapter, we urge critical reflection on the impacts of removing access to diagnostic imaging and the message that 'imaging findings don't matter' in all cases, though we do endorse the adoption of imaging guidelines for identifying those in whom imaging is unlikely to change clinical intervention.

Pain as a biopsychosocial phenomenon

The currently most widely accepted model for understanding the experience of pain is usually referred to as the biopsychosocial (BPS) model. Originally described by George Engel in the late 1970s, the model was intended to be: 1) a more person-centered approach to understanding health, illness and suffering; and 2) a successor to the prevailing biomedical model that had guided medical research for decades (if not centuries). Engel leveled criticism at the overly narrow view of purely biomedical understandings of health and illness, endorsing a model requiring clinicians to consider not *only* the biological components, but also the psychological and sociocultural (environment, politics, culture, interpersonal dynamics) components (Engel, 1977). Opponents argued the BPS model was too 'soft' an approach to medicine and would push practice back to a time when physicians were akin to spiritual healers. In some circles, the BPS model was clearly not amenable to scientific inquiry and certainly difficult to objectify, and thus it is not surprising that it was not until the late 1980s before it started to catch on in earnest in mainstream medicine. Some of the leading thinkers in pain research, including Ronald Melzack and Louis Gifford, were clearly influenced as evidenced by their Neuromatrix (Melzack, 1999) and Mature Organism (Gifford, 1998) models; both of which include prominent biopsychosocial elements. However, as often happens, Engel's vision of the biopsychosocial model as a means to facilitate an integrated understanding of concepts like pain (as well as any other state of health or illness) has been often reduced to distinct dimensions (biology, psychology, sociology) owing largely to the need for definable academic disciplines. That is, while most clinicians we know would endorse a biopsychosocial understanding of pain, when asked about it they will still speak in terms of assessing the biological, the psychological, and the social aspects of pain as though they are distinct siloes of inquiry.

In comparison to purely biomedical approaches, the biopsychosocial approach is certainly a desirable move forward in clinical reasoning, however it still falls slightly short. While considering all domains is valuable, the concept that they are separate is artificial; there is no psychology *without* biology, and there is no biology *or* psychology *without* being driven by society, culture and environment. The Venn diagram in Figure 1.2 shows the biopsychosocial model, with the concept of being human in the middle where these three domains overlap and are arguably inseparable. Even the radar plot framework we describe in this book remains arguably too reductionistic, in that we

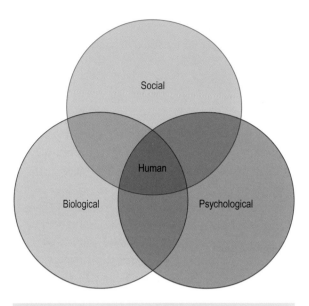

Figure 1.2
The Venn diagram of the biopsychosocial model, with the concept of being human in the middle where these three domains overlap and are arguably inseparable.

will not dive deeply into the intimate interactions that very likely exist between the domains. Partly, this is because the evidence to understand what those inter-actions look like is in its infancy, and partly because at some point we need to put boundaries around a clini-cal framework to make it useable.

If you've been paying attention so far, you may be wondering how to assess pain, how assessment should lead to treatment, and may even be wonder-ing, why bother, given the complexity of the phe-nomenon. To be clear, it's not an easy answer, but we've created and will describe a framework for clinical reasoning that appears to make a complex condition such as pain easier to understand and manage. The theory and framework can be illus-trated by returning to our earlier example of under-standing the experience of someone with their eyes closed who is swaying back and forth slowly. In iso-lation, it's hard to know exactly what's happening.

But, by considering multiple sources of informa-tion, you will get closer and closer to zeroing in on the true nature of the patient's experience. Do you hear music? Do you see earphones? Are other peo-ple doing the same thing? How old is this person? Are they alone? What are they wearing? What time of day is it? What do you already know about this person? All of these are things that you can discern mostly automatically and without much conscious thought – you haven't yet even asked them what they're doing. But, by considering multiple, easily accessible, and potentially rich sources of informa-tion simultaneously, you've begun the process of triangulating their experience. If you translate this to the experience of pain, you will likely, intuitively, conduct a similar pseudo-interpretive analysis to understand your patient's experience: How old is this person? What behaviors are they demonstrating? Do you see any signs of damage or injury? Perhaps their sex (or the sex with which they identify), cultural background, or ethnicity will factor in. Maybe you've seen this person before and so have some sense of their past experiences and a baseline for how they respond to pain. Again, all of these data are being 'sampled' before you've asked your first question. In a nutshell, this is the paradigm we'll be endorsing through this book, demonstrating how your intui-tion can be supplemented with rigorously designed but simple to apply clinical tools to get you progres-sively closer to understanding not only your patient's pain experience, but more importantly, what strate-gies for management are likely to be most effective.

Couching the subjective experience of pain within a philosophical framework for treatment decisions

Prior to embarking on a detailed description of the philosophy and framework of *Assess, Predict, Treat*, it is prudent to pause momentarily and discuss in at least broad terms, the nature of evidence, knowledge, and how those are created and used in medical and rehabilitation science. Germane to this discussion, and the framework, is an overview of how new knowledge is created, and how it applies to something as vague as the experience of pain. Perhaps in doing so, we will also start to glimpse the nature of what are sometimes loud and occasionally even hostile discords, debates, and disagreements between clinicians or researchers around the way pain *ought* to be approached and addressed.

Epistemic philosophies attempt to describe the nature of knowledge (new or old), that is, how do we know what we know? Where did that come from? And whose purpose is that knowledge serving? Much of epistemology is also rooted in the study of reality, also termed ontology, which is focused on understanding how we know what is real, and if what is real to me is similarly real to you. Here we describe three broad schools of thought on the nature of knowledge.

Post-positivism

The first one to address is post-positivism. Emerging out of the *positivism* (the search for universal laws and truths) movement, post-positivism became the dominant approach to conducting, interpreting, and understanding science in the last third of the twentieth century. Where positivism was based on a theory that there is a single universal reality and that through adequately rigorous data collection and analysis we can sample, uncover, and understand the laws that govern that reality (and thereby perfectly predict things like cause-and-effect), post-positivism accepted that a single universal reality exists but that we can never fully grasp it. In other words, we can conduct good science and become fairly confident that X causes Y, but we can never be 100% confident in that relationship. It recognizes that reality, and our ability to grasp it, is more fragile and tenuous than the positivists would have hoped. This is why most research studies, those that are focused on finding cause-and-effect relationships, will report things like probability (p) values and confidence limits – we're never 100% confident that a difference or relationship exists, but we're generally satisfied when we can, with 95% confidence, state a difference is likely to exist. Not perfect, but a more accurate representation of post-positivism, e.g. if we *disprove* enough *alternative* hypotheses (with at least 95% confidence) then over time we become increasingly close to the true nature of the *association, difference, or effect*.

If you've ever interpreted a sample size as 'too small' or considered the generalizability of findings from a research study (to what extent do these findings likely apply to different contexts and to the patient or patients that I typically work with), then you've engaged in post-positivistic thinking, inasmuch as you believe there is a single universal reality out there even if we can't be 100% certain we know what that is. There's a very important aspect to this line of thinking: that there are very few facts, laws, or truths in post-positivism. And this is probably a good first stop on our journey to understanding the nature of evidence especially when it comes to applying it to something as nebulous as pain.

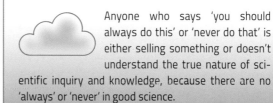
Anyone who says 'you should always do this' or 'never do that' is either selling something or doesn't understand the true nature of scientific inquiry and knowledge, because there are no 'always' or 'never' in good science.

Constructivism

On the far opposite end of the epistemic continuum are the constructivist (or constructionist) paradigms. Constructivism, as a means of understanding knowledge, posits that there is no such thing as a single universal truth, rather there are infinite realities unique to each of us. For example, if I were to write that I'm currently sitting in a chair while typing this sentence, you can very likely conjure a mental representation of a chair. While it's highly unlikely that you will conjure the exact same image of a chair as the one I'm sitting in, that itself is not necessarily a different reality. We both understand the concept of a chair. However, constructivists would say that if you and I were both looking at the same chair, at the same time, the ways in which we experience or understand that chair would be different. If you and I were to try and describe our understandings of that chair, our lived experiences of observing that chair, or the meaning of that chair, it would likely be different in a way that goes beyond simply using language differently.

In another example, a post-positivist would likely believe that she could prove all swans in the world are white: if she could only sample every single swan that currently exists and as long as they are all white, problem answered. Constructivists however would be likely to state something along the lines of: it doesn't matter what you've found because you and I interpret and experience 'white swan' differently, so your reality is not the same as mine. In constructivist-driven research then, concepts like probabilities, confidence, or generalizability are meaningless. As a constructivist researcher, all I'd be interested in is *your* experience of something, and I fully accept that what I'm hearing is *my* interpretation of *your* experience, which is what then gets reported in a research paper to the extent that *I* can use written language to adequately describe *my* understanding of *your* experience. There is much we can take from constructivist paradigms in pain research and management, including that the experiencing person's narrative about their experience is indeed the closest thing we can get to a gold standard for pain (or any other experience for that matter, hearkening back to Daniel Gilbert's comments earlier), and that my interpretation of your narrative cannot be separated from my own lived experiences of pain. Therefore, my

understanding is going to be an imperfect representation of what you're telling me. Once you start to wrap your head around that, then it becomes slightly easier to understand those times when, despite applying the best research evidence available, the patient in front of you still does not appear to be getting 'better'. What exactly 'better' means in the context of *this* patient with *that* pain experience is a topic we encourage you to stop and reflect upon during your next clinical encounter.

Critical realism

Fortunately, there are several in-between points along the epistemic continuum that represent some kind of intermingling of these two extremes. One that we will harness here is termed *critical realism*. To say that critical realism is simply a blend of post-positivism and constructivism would miserably fail to appreciate the complexities of these schools of thought. But for our purposes, that might be a good way for the novice learner to start thinking. Critical realists will argue that a single universal reality exists through the combination of the empirical, the actual, and the real, but only one of those can we observe. In this case, the *empirical* reality is that which can be observed and measured, our 'lived world' so to speak, that we can grasp and describe. The *actual* reality is what exists around us (or the researcher) but is not (easily) observable, and *real* reality is something largely untouchable by science or direct personal experience but is a sort of deeper layer of causal mechanisms that drive the actual and empirical.

Do you see how this attempt to blend complex schools of thought can quickly burden our minds with the different philosophies of knowledge? Perhaps it is best to stick with the notion that, from the critical realist perspective, ideas and constructs are not necessarily fixed, but they are 'real'. Where Newton could be most easily understood as a positivist who gave us universal laws of motion and those laws could be used to predict the precise time it would take for an apple to hit the ground, a critical realist would say that even this is not a universal truth in that our experiences of the apple or the ground are likely different and may change over time. So, while we can come up with a formula that generally works to predict certain observations, this itself is simply an observable effect of a more complex set of mechanisms governed by some unobservable 'real' reality. We will draw several notions from critical realism including the idea that empirical observations can help us understand an unobservable reality (such as a patient's actual pain experience) but that we can never fully grasp it, and at best we can only measure the empirical surface layer of a complex multi-layer causal arrangement. We will also borrow the critical realist position that ideas, values, and beliefs are also real things and, if done properly, can be measured in an accurate *enough* way to allow us to at least predict certain events such as whether our patient is likely to recover spontaneously (with or without our help) or is at risk for poor recovery, though always appreciating that those realities are not fixed.

We will use critical realist thinking to frame our conversations about pain and how best to understand it. We will start from a position that pain and the experience thereof is a real thing even if we cannot see it, touch it, or even fully understand all of the mechanisms driving it (analogous to the 'real reality'). We will further accept that the patient is themselves able to experience the pain through some form of interoception (Box 1.3) necessarily viewed through their own unique lens of life experiences, genetic vulnerabilities, culture, expectation, and a host of other definable or undefinable influences that as clinicians we can approximate with sound assessment but never fully grasp (analogous to the 'actual reality'). We will finally accept the 'epistemic reality' as the junction where clinician

> **Box 1.3** Interoception
>
> Interoception can be most easily defined as the ability to sense the internal state of one's body. This does not however necessarily mean that a person can: 1) interpret it properly; and 2) describe it to someone else. We all have it, though likely don't think too much about the internal state of our body when things are all in good order. It's when something 'feels off' or is in a state of some degree of trouble that this ability to sense what's happening on the inside, whether consciously or unconsciously (e.g. 'I can't put my finger on it, but something just isn't right') becomes important.

and patient can meet and develop some shared understanding of the experience. This will require sound measurement, clinical assessment and observation, Socratic questioning, therapeutic rapport, and a process of interpretivist reasoning drawn partly from constructivism. Figure 1.3 shows this in a diagrammatic way.

The intent of this short section is not to jostle your brain or draw the ire of followers of any of these epistemic philosophies. Our intent rather is to highlight the fragility of scientific knowledge, and especially the fact that when we try to apply traditional ways of thinking about knowledge to something as messy as a human being, it is highly unlikely that we're going to find *any* universal truths or laws to govern our thinking. However, again borrowing from the critical realist perspective, if we make enough observations and interpret them according to our own world views, there is a good chance that we will start to better understand the complex workings of a patient's experience of pain and provide us as clinicians with enough direction to craft person-centered (and patient-partnered) intervention strategies.

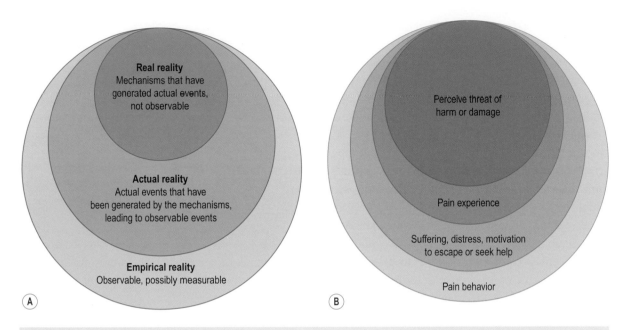

Figure 1.3
A simple diagrammatic representation of critical realist thought. **(A)** In this philosophy, a 'real' reality exists in which resides the mechanisms that drive our experiences, but despite being real cannot be directly observed or measured. The actual reality is the result of those mechanisms, and can be experienced but not measured. The epistemic reality is the observable manifestation of those experiences, and which, if the tools exist, can be measured. **(B)** An example of how critical realist thought can be mapped onto the experience of pain. Here we believe the perception of harm or damage is 'real', but cannot be directly grasped by either the experiencer (patient) or outside observer (clinician). The patient can however experience pain and suffering and this becomes their 'actual' reality, though it remains somewhat invisible to the observer. Where the patient and clinician meet is with the outward behaviors indicating pain, which in our analogy could be observed, maybe even measured, and will be called the empirical reality of pain.

With this brief background in mind, we now turn to a critical reflection on the value and limitations of clinical research, such that the subsequent sections of this book and the reasons we are endorsing a framework focused on rich assessment, triangulation, and phenotyping (rather than strict subgrouping) begin to make more sense.

Clinical research: value and limitations

As will be described in Chapter 2, the philosophy of *Assess, Predict, Treat* is centered around an approach to clinical reasoning that makes it more likely that the right treatment is provided at the right time for the right patient towards the right outcome(s). This presents a slight challenge for strong advocates of exclusively evidence-based treatment decisions, insofar as evidence gleaned from traditional randomized controlled trials (RCTs) rarely allow consideration of the unique characteristics of individual patients or those unobservable actual and real components of human experience. While rigorous RCTs are often viewed as the gold standard for establishing cause-and-effect, they require acceptance of the assumption that with large enough samples and true randomization, the unique characteristics of people that might otherwise affect their response to treatment (often referred to as 'confounders') are equally distributed between groups and therefore 'washed out' and rendered unimportant when comparing group averages. In other words, a good randomization procedure should lead to equal distribution of confounders (those extraneous things that affect research results) between the comparator groups. While this thinking may work well for genetically similar agricultural crop research (an approach endorsed by statistician and geneticist R.A. Fisher in the early 1900s), it is more problematic for research on humans where unique individual traits are important. Such traits are not likely to be perfectly replicated, let alone even similar, in two people that find themselves in opposite comparator groups of a clinical trial. It is therefore worth remembering that RCTs and the knowledge they provide, while offering *some* evidence of cause-and-effect, are based largely on group means of usually fairly homogenous subsamples rather than providing an indication of how each individual participant in the study responded. Those subsamples are themselves part of a much larger patient population, and all of this may be rarely applicable to the particular patient sitting in front of you. In fact, most research findings will report group means to one level of precision greater than the data that were collected (e.g. the mean of 2 and 3 on a 10-point numeric rating scale is 2.5) meaning that no single patient in the entire study will have actually fallen directly on the mean. Keep in mind that a mean, the average of all numbers, is only a mean because the people (or their scores) fell equal distances on either side of that number. So this begs the question: to whom, if anyone, are the results of this type of clinical research applicable?

This is of course not to suggest that sound empirical research is unimportant – we are, after all, researchers ourselves. However, our years of clinical experience combined with years of research have led

to a consistent finding: *no intervention will work for everyone, but it seems every intervention will work for someone.* To take an extreme example, a slap in the face may be the right intervention for the right person at the right time within the right context (though we do not endorse this approach, and you are unlikely to find any trials on the effectiveness of face slapping). Your challenge as a clinician is to first identify the pieces of the puzzle that define the person, then figure out how they fit together to form a 'picture' of the best course of treatment. And, if they are not responding to this approach, rethink the pieces of the puzzle and start over. It could be that your measurement tools need calibrating, or your intervention strategy needs tweaking, rather than blaming the patient for his/her failure to respond to the plan of care.

The next time you review an RCT that found negative results (no difference between groups), look for evidence describing the distribution of scores between the comparison groups (maybe a figure or table); chances are there will be people in the active group who did respond favorably, and some who got worse or had no change. Similarly, there will be some in the control group who responded and some who got worse. If only 10% of the active treatment group responded better than the control, then most research designs would likely report no significant mean difference by virtue of the way such data are analyzed, and the treatment would be considered ineffective. But what of those 10% who responded favorably? Most research designs are ill-equipped to allow these types of *post hoc* subgroup analyses, but clinicians conduct 'subgroup analyses' every day, the subgroup in this case being the individual patient. Wouldn't you like to know when you see the 1 in 10 who should actually respond to that treatment?

The point so far is that research evidence should be accessed and leveraged for facilitating clinical decisions but should not be the only source of information used to decide treatment pathways. We often say to novice clinicians that if you were to only practice in accordance with rigorous clinical trials, then not only would your treatment options be terribly limited, but if you were to look back over the course of your entire career you would likely be able to say that, *on average*, the people you treated tended to do better than those who received no treatment or an alternate treatment. Surely most can strive for better than average.

We believe that optimal care comes in the form of sound assessment and prediction of the natural and clinical course of a patient's health condition. In an era of personalized medicine, there is no reason that rehabilitation for musculoskeletal pain should receive any less attention. The term *personalized medicine* is most often used in the context of genetic screening to identify profiles of patients (or phenotypes) who may respond with more or less effect to pharmaceutical treatments (Box 1.4).

Box 1.4 Personalized medicine

An example of personalized medicine can be found from recent guidelines suggesting that around 20 to 30% of patients with pain may have a genetic defect involving one of three major cytochrome P450 enzymes and so cannot effectively metabolize certain opioids. Opioids must be metabolized by the liver to become active, which means that those who are unable to efficiently metabolize opioids would need much higher doses than rapid metabolizers to get the same effect. This work helps us to consider the importance of understanding the value of the cytochrome P450 gene for discriminating between *high* and *low* opioid metabolizers.

So, what are the 'personalized rehabilitation' markers we should be exploring for prescribing conservative therapies? Here, we take the concept of clinical phenotypes and present a new framework for creating patient profiles that facilitate *right care, right patient, right time*. While we are not ignoring research-based techniques or tools that are generally limited to the laboratory, we are intentionally favoring clinical techniques and tools that are widely available to the average clinician. Therefore, you won't read that we suggest tissue biopsy, advanced imaging techniques like functional MRI, or genotyping be performed on every patient walking through your clinic door. However, some of this may not be far off, and it is important we increase our awareness of research-based techniques and tools (some of which stems from our own work) as new findings from such advancements may result in change of clinical practice. For example, researchers collaborating between Sweden and California recently published a proof-of-concept study demonstrating how they used a smartphone camera to sequence the genome of tumor cells (Kühnemund et al., 2017), opening the door for potential future advancements in rapid smartphone-based genotyping of humans. Perhaps the next version of this text will indeed include more biological assays completed at the point of care within the list of tools available to everyday clinicians.

The question of course then becomes: what evidence base are we able to draw upon to provide the recommendations in this book? Here we turn to the current directions in the field of evidence-informed medicine/rehabilitation (EIM or EIR) that considers the best patient-centered decisions based on research evidence, provider experience, and patient values (to the extent they can be understood), and where needed, in an interdisciplinary fashion. Where it's available, we will cite research evidence from which the statements in this book are drawn, but where it's unavailable, the suggestions will be based on our own experiences and opinions as clinicians, patient advocates, academics, and our own lived experiences as humans dedicated to helping people in pain. This approach is necessitated as we adopt a critical realist approach to understanding pain, disability, and rehabilitation, and the consideration of research evidence, clinician experience and patient values is the first example of triangulation of several more to come throughout this book.

References

Bennett, C. M., Baird, A. A., Miller, M. B., et al., 2009. Neural correlates of interspecies perspective taking in the post-mortem Atlantic Salmon: An argument for multiple comparisons correction. Available at: http://prefrontal.org/files/posters/Bennett-Salmon-2009.pdf.

Engel, G. L., 1977. The need for a new medical model: a challenge for biomedicine. *Science* 196 (4286):129–36.

Cohen, M., Quintner, J., Buchanan, D., et al., 2011. Stigmatization of patients with chronic pain: the extinction of empathy. *Pain Medicine* 12 (11):1637–43.

Gifford, L., 1998. Pain, the tissues and the nervous system: a conceptual model. *Physiotherapy* 84 (1):27–36.

Gilbert, D., 2006. *Stumbling on happiness.* Harper Press; London.

Kühnemund, M., Qingshan, W., Evangelia Darai, E., et al., 2017. Targeted DNA sequencing and *in situ* mutation analysis using mobile phone microscopy. *Nature Communications* 8: 13913.

Melzack, R., 1999. From the gate to the neuromatrix. *Pain* Suppl 6:S121–6.

Rhodes, L. A., McPhillips-Tangum, C. A., Markham, C., et al., 1999. The power of the visible: the meaning of diagnostic tests in chronic back pain. *Social Science & Medicine* 48 (9):1189–203.

Slade, S. C., Molloy, E., Keating, J. L., 2009. Stigma experienced by people with nonspecific chronic low back pain: a qualitative study. *Pain Medicine* 10 (1):143–54.

2

The Assess, Predict, Treat Framework

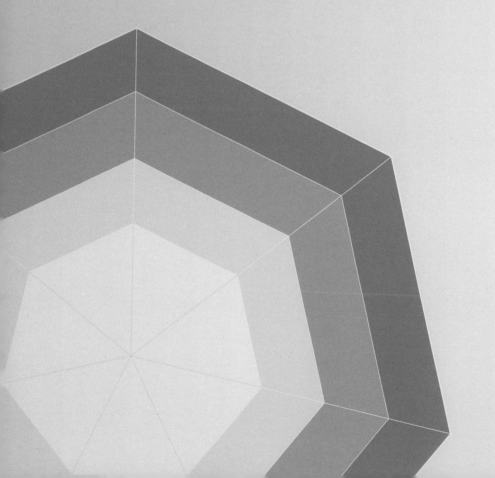

The concept of *Assess, Predict,* and *Treat* doesn't sound particularly innovative at first mention. In fact, it should seem like a common-sense approach to managing your patient's reported complaints or observed 'problems', which is exactly what it is. Conduct a sound, comprehensive, critically-informed and clinically-relevant assessment of the patient (including documented history, subjective narrative, consider results from a wide variety of available clinical tools and objective clinical tests); use those findings to predict the likelihood that the patient will: a) improve on their own, or b) respond to a particular treatment; and then treat them according to your assessment and prediction. However, while it seems like common sense, our experience is that many clinicians find this reasoning process and application difficult. Perhaps this is not surprising, especially as we contrast what is increasingly known about the experiences of pain and disability (and the biopsychosocial complexities thereof) and what the more biomedical approaches commonly prioritize in healthcare training programs. In order to properly implement an *APT framework,* clinicians must first possess considerable knowledge on the choice, application and interpretation of clinical assessment tools (including effective interview skills, use and interpretation of standardized self-report tools, and clinician-administered clinical tests), be able to combine and use those findings to mentally construct a multidimensional profile of the patient, identify important patterns in their presentation, have an up-to-date working knowledge on the prognostic and theranostic utility of a variety of clinical variables (assuming the evidence exists), and then be able to match treatment decisions to what is often a very complex clinical picture. Even the most seasoned clinicians have difficulty applying these principles in a coherent and logical way, often falling back on early-career training, heuristics, and intuition when choosing the 'best course' of action for their patients.

Facilitating clinical reasoning

The APT framework has been developed to make these processes more manageable for the busy clinician. It won't take all of the intuition or 'gut feeling' type of work out of a clinical encounter, nor will we ignore the value of that previous experience or clinician intuition. Further, no clinical framework will be right 100% of the time and your own reasoning will remain an important component of any clinical interaction and decision. By choosing and applying a select set of meaningful clinical evaluation techniques, using the results to create a visual representation of the patient's profile, and comparing that to what *is* currently known about prognosis, theranosis, and treatment options, APT can make a messy and complex picture more interpretable and lead to treatment decisions that are rational, justified, and easily adaptable to the patient's response (or lack thereof).

It is not a new method of classification or subgrouping of patients into distinct categories. In fact, the concept of creating a multidimensional profile represents a departure from the practice of creating distinct clinical subgroups that was a primary focus of research in the musculoskeletal pain field through much of the 2000s and early 2010s. We believe a departure is necessary as subgrouping assumes humans can and do fall neatly into distinct categories, but as clinicians will know, this is rarely the simple case. Many classifications in the 'clinical prediction rule' types of approaches involved identifying the presence (and sometimes magnitude) of three, four, or more signs or symptoms to consider a patient 'positive' on the scale. Anecdotally this is problematic as many patients may satisfy some of the criteria but not all, leaving clinicians with more confusion than clarity about how to defend their treatment choices. Moreover, as readers get more comfortable in a critical realist thinking paradigm, it should be noted that the creation of subgroups is dependent on the variables that a particular research group chose to capture (how that research group chose to sample the 'empirical reality'). As a result, the rules of classification algorithms are necessarily limited to *those* variables *that* group of researchers thought were important while excluding all others. Here again we come back to our triangulation concept from Chapter 1 (described further below), that treatment decisions must be made on the basis of a combination of evidence, your own clinical experience/intuition, and the values and expectations of the patient in front of you.

To provide a concrete example of that last paragraph, consider this scenario: a researcher wants to determine whether the very popular Pain Catastrophizing Scale (PCS) identifies different subgroups of people with neck pain. Since we already know that the PCS shows fairly consistent relationships with the commonly used Neck Disability Index (NDI), we can already tell you how this would go without looking at a lick of data. A *latent class analysis* (LCA, type of cluster analysis) using scores on the PCS from a sample of people with neck pain would identify three subgroups: one who scores low across the board on all items, one who scores mid-range, and a smaller group that scores high. That's the most common cluster solution for most interval-level data analyzed with LCA especially with sample sizes below about 200-300 (Walton et al., 2015; Walton et al., 2016; Walton et al., 2013; Sterling et al., 2010). And of course, we can predict that NDI scores would be different across those three clusters, and those in the low category would have better outcome X (let's say, return to work) than would those in the high cluster. In fact, our collaborative research groups have identified this general pattern a few times now, using things like pressure pain detection threshold (PPDT) and the Brief Illness Perceptions Questionnaire (BIPQ) (Fig. 2.1).

Of course, you could raise the 'fancy bar' even higher by tossing multiple variables into your analysis – let's go with PPDT and PCS scores to stick with our current example. The results will almost certainly suggest different categories exist based on the combinations of these two tools – one cluster with low PCS scores but heightened pain sensitivity, one with low

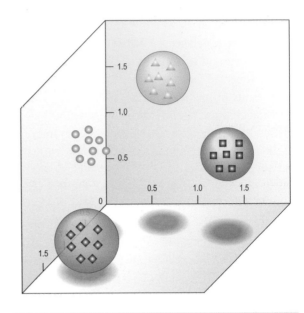

Figure 2.1

A diagrammatic representation of latent class analysis. Statistical techniques are used to identify clusters of patients that show similar variance or associations between two or more clinical signs, and are distinct from the magnitude of variance or association in other clusters.

pain sensitivity but high PCS scores, and every combination in between. But the question becomes: are those the *right* subgroups? What happens if someone else comes along and instead uses cold pain threshold (CPT) and the Depression, Anxiety and Stress scale (DASS), and again creates a method to subgroup and again (as expected) shows that their groups are different based on NDI scores or something else. Evidence is fairly clear on that last part: *the higher one rates on 'terribleness' scale A, the higher they'll also rate on 'terribleness' scale B* regardless of what that construct has been called (or whether that's even useful information). What happens when a brand-new scale comes along that's *better* than either the PCS or the DASS? We would have to start from square one on our subgrouping research – it's a never-ending cycle with no definitive conclusions on the horizon.

Then of course there is a multitude of other questions to ask each time a subgrouping algorithm is created: For what is it useful (e.g. treatment decisions or prognosis)? Whose interest does it serve (e.g. your own, the patient's, or the funder's)? Who might this rule unintentionally harm? What happens when a patient does not fit the rule? What other sources of information could be used to arrive at the same conclusion? Do interventions that target those variables lead to improved clinical outcomes over other more standard care approaches? Are these variables more mechanistic (are they actually telling us something directly about the patient) or are they better viewed as proxies for other mechanisms (i.e. are there confounders at work here)?

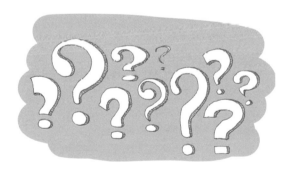

To drive home this point in an admittedly facetious way, we could very likely create subgroups of patients with neck pain based on whether they ate a hot breakfast, a cold breakfast, or no breakfast at all. It wouldn't surprise us in the least if NDI scores were different between the no breakfast and the hot breakfast groups, and we could then postulate about mechanisms for years to come. Do those who get to eat a hot breakfast have fewer dependents (children) at home? Are they in a different socioeconomic class than those who ate no breakfast at all? Do those

who ate no breakfast also live in an area commonly referred to as a 'food desert'? Are they dealing with more daily life stressors? Are they lacking some key nutrient for recovery otherwise found in some hot breakfasts? Regardless, this type of approach to creating subgroups (which is more common than you may realize) offers little guidance on treatment decisions.

Profiling or *phenotyping* on the other hand allows far more flexibility in clinical reasoning and decision-making. Through the use of concepts like triangulation and graphical plotting (discussed below and in Chapter 3), new evidence can be immediately incorporated into the clinical reasoning process without requiring the whole cycle of practice-to-evidence-to-practice to start anew each time. The APT framework places high value on sound assessment and evaluation techniques, both through effective interpersonal communication and appropriate clinical tests, with a belief that prognosis and treatment ought to naturally flow from assessment findings. Does the patient appear to have a good handle on their pain problem in terms of beliefs and expectations? Then cognitive approaches probably aren't necessary. But that doesn't preclude emotional pathology that should be addressed. In this way, the creation of a patient-by-patient profile allows more diverse, nuanced, and targeted care decisions without any dramatic increase in clinician (or patient) burden. In fact, when used properly, we find the APT framework not only improves clinical decision making but also reduces clinician burden and improves patient satisfaction.

Assess

In the APT model, every assessment or evaluation procedure is chosen with purpose and sound reasoning. The goal of the patient assessment is to construct a *profile* that, if needed, can be graphically displayed on a radar plot (or any other type of plot for that matter – if you like bar charts, use a bar chart). The graphical depiction should then point the clinician towards appropriate treatment decisions. The current iteration of the radar plot (Fig. 2.2) is a seven-point arrangement that includes the following domains: **Nociceptive/Physiological, Peripheral Neuropathic, Central Nociplastic, Emotional/Affective, Cognitive/Belief, Socioenvironmental,** and **Sensorimotor Dysintegration**.

As of this writing, we believe that these seven points capture enough of the important domains of the experience of pain and disability for clinicians to understand their patient's experience, and should lead to different targeted treatment decisions. However, the intention is not to 'sell' the radar plot – like every component of the APT framework, it is fluid and can (and will) be expanded/reduced/revised as new evidence emerges. The important contribution of such a plot is that it allows

organization of findings and facilitates interpretation of complex conditions, giving structure to recognizing our patients' clinical patterns and profiles. It is intended as a mid-way point between the art (intuition) and science (empiricism) of clinical practice without valorizing either one. It is intended to provide a means to interpret information without necessitating the collection of only 'hard numbers' in its creation.

Creation of the plot involves clinical triangulation of each patient's location on the domains, starting with or even before the clinical interview. In many ways, every question asked, or behavior observed, during the interview can be considered a data point in your clinical test, in that the answers to those questions should be leading to shifts in the probability that any of the seven domains are contributing to the patient's pain or disability. Similarly, every patient-reported measure and clinical observation should also

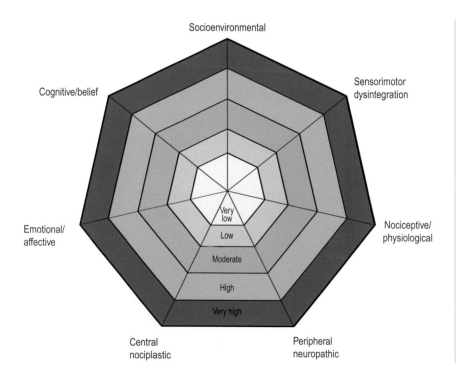

Figure 2.2
The current seven-point radar plot, with labels describing different drivers of the pain experience. The seven points have been chosen with intention, out of a belief that assessment and intervention strategies should be different between each. The relative contributions of each driver have been described descriptively (very low to very high) rather than quantitatively, as evidence is frequently changing.

be serving the purpose of constructing the patient profile. Assessment tools and techniques are chosen for their empirical support as discriminatory tests, with high value placed on low burden/high value tests that provide rich information (e.g. a single patient-reported scale may simultaneously strengthen the profile in one domain while reducing other domains). For this to happen, clinicians must be familiar with proper selection, application, and interpretation of available tests, as simply administering a scale without critical thought for its selection and interpretation is not good enough. Clinicians should, at the very least, possess knowledge of meaningful cut scores (or know how to find them) and ideally would also have some degree of knowledge on the discriminatory accuracy (validity) of those scores (e.g. sensitivity, specificity, positive or negative likelihood ratios). This way, clinicians can not only interpret the individual responses on a scale (which they all ought to do), but also the overall summed scores, and decide how much of a shift in the domain of the radar plot occurs as a result.

The concept of triangulation also fits with our critical realist perspective from Chapter 1. While we accept that *at best* all we can sample is the empirical reality of the patient, by looking at that reality from multiple viewpoints and perspectives we can get closer to grasping the *actual reality* of that patient's experience. The *real reality* likely remains out of reach and, we argue, is not necessary for forming a therapeutic alliance and a patient-partnered intervention plan. We believe however that moving closer to the actual reality of the patient's experience, an experience they themselves may have difficulty expressing or verbalizing, represents an important step forward in the evolution of clinical pain intervention.

Assessment in this framework is also not limited to the traditional domain of conservative rehabilitation providers. Findings from appropriate and targeted diagnostic imaging, blood work, or electrophysiological studies (as examples) can, and in some cases should, also inform the construction of the radar plot profile for selected patients. As with many of the tests described herein, this may require a new skillset to allow clinicians to appropriately request and interpret findings from assessment tools with which they're not familiar. Additionally, this requires an understanding of the relative value, burden, and limitations of even high-precision diagnostic procedures. As an example, it has become rather popular to denounce the value of diagnostic imaging in what are often deemed uncomplicated cases of low back pain owing to data from observational cohort studies that suggest most findings are not strongly related to clinical presentation and that many findings are present in asymptomatic populations. However, there are most certainly times when the ability to look inside the body may be warranted, perhaps even critical, to better understand a patient's experience and the drivers thereof. Consider that evidence from cross-sectional studies has shown that pathology is associated with some low back pain, even more so in those with a genetic vulnerability to producing excess pro-inflammatory cytokines in response to intervertebral disc herniation (at least in rats) (Wang et al., 2017; Tran et al., 2014; Tian et al., 2016). This is another example of the value of considering multiple sources of data: perhaps in the majority of people a lumbar or cervical disc herniation is asymptomatic, but when present in those who *also* express certain genetic traits, the combination of those two do show a relationship to pain. If this line of research extends to humans, and there's no reason to believe it will not, we once again could be left with treatment decisions that are made with incomplete information if old ways of categorical thinking about spinal pain and imaging are maintained. The use of triangulation and radar plots should protect against premature rejection of diagnostic, assessment or treatment strategies by allowing new evidence to be integrated as it becomes available. We anticipate, as an example, that determining the role of imaging in low back pain (and other common, yet equally enigmatic musculoskeletal conditions) is important as it could help identify patients belonging to distinct phenotypes that may be amenable to more informed and practical management approaches. A themed message in this book remains that astute clinicians are encouraged to consider all sources of information when selecting appropriate evaluation procedures for the patient in front of them.

Predict

This is the 'future telling' part of the process. Following from the sound assessment, the next logical questions to ask are: does this patient require treatment, and if yes, then what treatment is most likely to lead to a positive outcome? This is a question that must again be asked on a patient-by-patient basis. In the case of a favorable prognosis, the APT framework endorses an arm's length approach to care: provide advice and education, and follow-up at a reasonable later time to ensure recovery is occurring as expected. In fact, we are rather emphatic about the idea that, where the natural course (prognosis) is determined to be favorable, early interventions should be *avoided* as we risk contributing to *iatrogenic disability*. Iatrogenic disability is the term given to the phenomenon of making a patient feel more disabled than they may otherwise be through an insistence that they require care – 'I must be more disabled than I thought, why else would this health expert be telling me I really need care?'

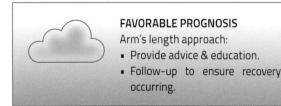

FAVORABLE PROGNOSIS
Arm's length approach:
- Provide advice & education.
- Follow-up to ensure recovery occurring.

Where prognosis is unfavorable or deemed to be improvable through appropriate treatment, we then shift focus from prognosis to *theranosis*, or the prediction of outcome given the introduction of a particular therapy (theranosis = 'therapy + prognosis'). Knowing both of these things (prognosis and theranosis) requires sound understanding of current evidence regarding normal recovery trajectories and the variables that may cause deviation (improving or slowing) of those trajectories.

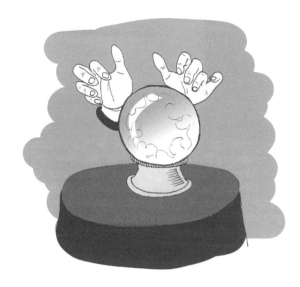

We are not selling the idea that prediction of the future is achievable (or even, practical). We fully recognize that predicting the future of recovery for a patient represents an imperfect science, not much different than predicting the weather or pork-belly futures. Central to the clinician's ability for predicting future events is the understanding of the natural course of a condition, many of which have been published (Fig. 2.3), and What variables may lead to deviation from those trajectories. The presence of some variables may hasten recovery while others may slow or even prevent it from occurring. Framing it in this way as 'What variables are present in my patient that may lead to a deviation from rapid recovery?' is a sound way to conceptualize the problem and will

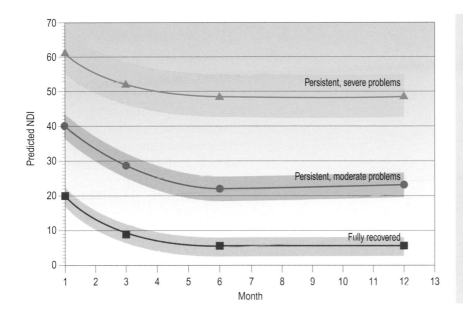

Figure 2.3
Sample of common recovery trajectories, adapted from those derived by Sterling et al. (2010) in people following acute whiplash. The 3-trajectory model is becoming consistent, though the shapes of those curves and proportions of patients in each tend to vary somewhat. When attempting to predict outcome, predicting as 'good' or 'bad' is too simplistic. Predictions should also include provision for those who recover but continue to experience mild to moderate problems.

only facilitate the development of a more informed plan of care (or referral). By additionally contemplating what *recovery* would look like for this patient, this kind of thinking provides a means to choose and establish meaningful clinical outcomes.

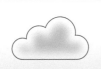

UNFAVORABLE PROGNOSIS
Remember – predisposed does not mean predestined.
Consider multimodal and interdisciplinary treatment, including physical rehabilitation with a focus on mobility and pain management strategies, pharmaceutical interventions, psychology (to address fear and anxiety and improve coping strategies), possibly occupational therapy, social work, or other disciplines as appropriate.

It is also worth noting here that new 'big data' capture (which is really just a bunch of small data points from a very large group of individual patients) and analytics approaches continue to improve prediction algorithms. In the absence of sound big data-based predictive algorithms (few of which currently exist), the APT model builds a prognostic and predictive platform from the current evidence on consistent risk factors for chronic pain and disability. However, as cloud computing and large databases continue to emerge, we expect the process of predicting outcomes to change and become more accurate. Now is the time to collect the right data on an individual level to ultimately inform big data efforts.

In the context of pain from injury, we will highlight, blend, and contextualize emerging models explaining chronicity. Several have been described, attempting to answer the question: why do some people get better following an injury while others do not? Some of the models informing the development of the APT framework are the:

1. Vlaeyen and Linton's Fear-Avoidance model

2. Various biomechanical or structural models

3. Stress-dysregulation models

4. Turk's Stress-Diathesis model

5. Gifford's Mature Organism Model

6. Melzack's Neuromatrix Model

7. Various Compensation Neurosis hypotheses

8. Our own Neuronal Interference model

PROGNOSIS UNKNOWN
- Difficult but requires further assessment and evaluation. Rx should flow naturally from there.
- Conservative rehabilitation with low-level pharmaceutical therapy likely suitable.
- Monitor closely to ensure recovery occurring.

A key component of professional development in this area is that clinicians become *critical consumers of knowledge*, developing the tools to critically interpret these models in the context of existing and new emerging evidence yet to come. These mechanistic models (described further in the following chapters) represent starting points for understanding the genesis of chronic pain and prediction thereof, but are not to be considered definitive end points providing a 'crystal ball' of a patient's future. With time and new research findings, it is anticipated that some of these models (and measures to support, or refute, the models) will be modified, combined, expanded, or removed. In some areas, such as acute neck or low back pain, prognostic algorithms or clinical prediction rules already exist. These should be appraised and those deemed to have reached an adequate level of rigor *and* are congruent with context and values of the population being treated should be implemented as screening tools for identifying patients at high risk. However, clinicians must recognize we are still far from understanding the mechanisms behind, or the prognostic value of, for example, a high pain

rating or post-traumatic hyperarousal. A well-worn idiom in research, ***association is not the same as causation***, should be observed here, meaning that intervention targeted at a specific risk factor *may not* have the effect you're expecting (Box 2.1). This has been demonstrated in recent large-scale trials, especially in traumatic neck pain (i.e. 'whiplash'), wherein interventions targeted at high-risk patients have not always led to better recoveries (Lamb et al., 2012). Other clinical trials *have* shown value from risk-targeted intervention in neck (Sterling et al., 2019) or low back pain (Hill et al., 2011), but even then the effects tend to be small. One interpretation is that *we cannot help these people*, but we would argue that a better interpretation is that high scores on a risk estimation tool are a proxy for some other process, rather than the culprit itself to be apprehended. In other words, while we are now fairly accurate at discriminating between the very high- and very low-risk patient, the mechanisms to explain that risk are still somewhat elusive.

Box 2.1 Association is not causation

A classic example of 'association is not causation' is the relationship between ice cream consumption in a community, and home robberies in that community. The more ice cream the community consumes, the more home robberies there are. One interpretation would be that eating ice cream causes people to subsequently start robbing homes, though that seems illogical. Another far more reasonable interpretation is that people both consume more ice cream, and that there tend to be more home robberies, when the weather is nice. In this case, the association may well exist, but causation cannot be assumed. The weather is a *confounding variable* in this example. There are very likely many, many examples of confounders, mediators and moderators in associations in pain research.

Treat

We suggest that the tools you use in combination should answer questions such as: what is the likelihood this person follows a normal recovery trajectory, and does this person need my care? However, we are encouraging all clinicians to beware of assuming that targeting the risk factors in clinical prediction algorithms will necessarily lead to improved outcomes. Both the *Assessment* and *Prediction* activities should interact to inform treatment decisions, not prediction alone.

This may come as unwanted news, but there are not a lot of rehabilitation or medical interventions, or even an intervention period, that enjoys consistent evidence of strong clinical short- or long-term effects for improving outcomes in acute or chronic pain. Where interventions have been studied in rigorous clinical trials, most, especially the conservative therapies, have been met with findings of small, moderate, or often even no significant effect. We will summarize these in the following chapters, but this is not meant to indicate we should do nothing for these patients. It needs to be noted here that clinical trials have *rarely* been able to stratify patients to the nuanced levels of unique clinical presentations and patterns that clinicians do almost intuitively. As such, in accordance with current evidence-informed practice models, clinicians should be aware of the evidence but not be paralyzed by it. Rather the evidence should be combined with clinical experience and patient values to arrive at a meaningful intervention strategy.

Rather than being beholden to *only* interventions that are supported by empirical evidence (of which, as we've said, there are very few), the APT philosophy encourages treatment decisions that flow naturally from assessment and prediction. If the first two have been conducted and interpreted properly, the following questions should make choosing the most appropriate treatment for an individual patient relatively easy:

1. What is/are the primary driver(s) of this patient's experience of pain or disability?

2. What is the likelihood that this patient's condition will improve without intervention?

3. To what intervention(s) is this patient most likely to respond?

1. What are the primary drivers?

The answer to question 1 comes from the radar plot and triangulation exercises. A useful analogy here might be of a sinking ship: in a ship with many holes, it makes sense to find and plug the biggest hole first, then move on to the next biggest and so on.

There are times this doesn't always hold true, as in the case where certain domains (e.g. cognitions) may be slightly smaller in magnitude than others (e.g. nociceptive), but theory and empiricism suggest that tackling nociceptive sources of pain without first, or at least simultaneously, addressing maladaptive and/or inaccurate cognitions will likely result in a smaller treatment effect. This highlights a key limitation in our knowledge at this time: do all domains deserve equal weighting when considering their contribution to the patient's experience of pain and disability? Currently this question is difficult to answer, but the above example using cognitions as an important driver to target does enjoy some degree of empirical support.

2. Is treatment indicated?

Question 2 is a prognostic question. As addressed above, that could be rephrased to ask: does this patient require treatment? In the case where prognosis appears to be favorable, the APT framework suggests a focus on advice and education, managing expectations, and infrequent follow-ups to ensure

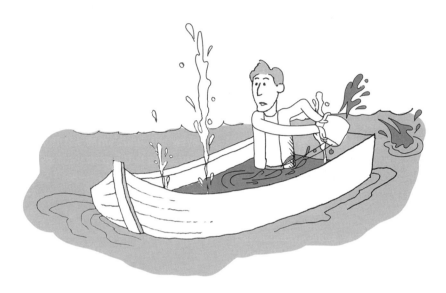

recovery is progressing as expected but to avoid over-treatment (i.e. an arm's length approach). As alluded to in the prior section, the intention is to avoid developing *iatrogenic disability*, or the genesis of disability due simply to receiving unnecessary treatment or diagnostic tests. Where prognosis is unfavorable (i.e. the patient is 'at risk'), the clinician should consider an additional two questions that are only answerable in tandem with the assessment findings: *at risk of what?* and *why?* Stating someone is 'at risk' of a poor outcome without having anything to do about it is not particularly helpful to anyone. This is admittedly an additional shortcoming of many prognostic algorithms and prediction rules currently available: they may function well to identify the at-risk patient but do little to provide treatment directions.

The question 'At risk of what?' is interesting to consider. At risk of continuing to experience (or at least report) pain beyond the expected recovery time? Perhaps at risk of continuing to rate high on disability scales? At risk of new psychopathology or physical comorbidity like depression or inactivity? How about at risk of not returning to work in a timely fashion, or continuing to receive wage indemnity benefits, or continuing to seek healthcare? There is a pervasive problem in this field that we cannot overlook, that being that the outcome being predicted has been highly inconsistent across a wide body of published research. Even where ongoing pain is the outcome, the thresholds for considering someone recovered has been inconsistent; some researchers may deem pain <3/10 as recovered, others 1/10, while still others accept only 0/10 pain to indicate recovery. This issue is currently being addressed on a global scale, and the Initiative for Measurement and Methods in Pain Clinical Trials (IMMPACT) group are one that have published core outcomes sets for pain clinical trials with the goal of greater standardization of outcomes and comparability across studies. It will likely be some time before we see adequately consistent outcomes to be able to answer some of these more difficult questions across all musculoskeletal conditions.

3. What treatment is indicated?

The answer to question 3, 'What treatment?', is largely theranostic in nature: to what type of treatment is this patient most likely to respond? The choice will be partly based on the radar plot (remember the sinking ship analogy) but should also consider, where possible, other influences on compliance and adherence to treatment recommendations. Things to consider include time, finances, access to resources/equipment, health literacy, lifestyle, interests, and patient values and goals. These are frequently included as components of health behavior change models drawn from health psychology literature (e.g. theory of planned behavior, health beliefs model, social learning theory) and clinicians are encouraged to become familiar with these well-established models of behavior. While several such theories exist, most boil down to this: can I do it?, and is it important? By exploring these questions with your patients, you may find techniques to improve adherence with treatment recommendations and optimize outcomes that cannot be found in published RCTs.

The APT model accepts and endorses that there is no one-size-fits-all approach to care, rather care decisions should be made considering the current best evidence (if it exists), the clinician's expertise and experience, and the patient's beliefs and values. Since traditional research studies are rarely designed to evaluate the effectiveness of care at an individual patient level, they are often not able to determine what type and intensity of treatment is right for Mrs. Jones sitting in front of you in the clinic. For this reason, the APT framework prioritizes sound assessment and prediction as the most important components of clinical intervention. Treatments should be customized to each patient based on these first two steps. We are trying to avoid getting caught in the 'when you have a hammer, everything looks like a nail' kind of thinking that tends to occur in clinicians following completion of a professional development course (think about the way your immediate practice changed the last time you took a treatment-focused course). Rather, this is a framework for clinical reasoning, that allows for and requires **curiosity, critical thinking**, and **creativity**.

Summary

In conclusion, the *Assess, Predict, Treat* framework for managing problems of musculoskeletal mobility deficits is not a radical departure from current routine clinical practice. It is more of a repackaging of what many already do, and what others would like to do better but are unsure of the 'how to'. By breaking the process of clinical decision making and pattern recognition into digestible steps it fosters skill development and an appreciation for the value and limitations of relying solely on research, clinician experience, or patient values in isolation. Importantly however, while breaking complex processes into manageable pieces is valuable for learning, eventually the processes must meld back together into a cohesive routine that may require new ways of thinking about patient interactions and requires ability to reflect upon one's own limitations in knowledge (and act upon those as part of lifelong learning). The term *critical consumer of knowledge* will inform our foci in this book, highlighting the importance of recognizing the value of knowledge from different sources but also understanding the limitations in what it can, and cannot, tell you.

References

Hill, J. C., Whitehurst, D. G., Lewis, M., et al., 2011. Comparison of stratified primary care management for low back pain with current best practice (STarT Back): a randomised controlled trial. *Lancet* 378 (9802):1560–71.

Lamb, S. E., Williams M. A., Williamson E. M., et al., 2012. Managing Injuries of the Neck Trial (MINT): a randomised controlled trial of treatments for whiplash injuries. *Health Technology Assessment* 16 (49):iii–iv, 1-141.

Sterling, M., Hendrikz, J., Kenardy, J., 2010. Compensation claim lodgement and health outcome developmental trajectories following whiplash injury: A prospective study. *Pain* 150 (1):22–8.

Sterling, M., Smeets, R., Keijzers, G., et al., 2019. Physiotherapist-delivered stress inoculation training integrated with exercise versus physiotherapy exercise alone for acute whiplash-associated disorder (StressModex): a randomised controlled trial of a combined psychological/physical intervention. *British Journal of Sports Medicine*: pii:bjsports-2018-100139.

Tian, Y., Yuan, W., Li, J., et al., 2016. TGFβ regulates Galectin-3 expression through canonical Smad3 signaling pathway in nucleus pulposus cells: implications in intervertebral disc degeneration. *Matrix Biology* 50:39–52.

Tran, C. M., Schoepflin, Z. R., Markova, D. Z., et al., 2014. CCN2 suppresses catabolic effects of interleukin-1β through α5β1 and αVβ3 integrins in nucleus pulposus cells: implications in intervertebral disc degeneration. *Journal of Biological Chemistry* 289 (11):7374–87.

Walton, D. M., Eilon-Avigdor, Y., Wonderham, M., et al., 2013. Exploring the clinical course of neck pain in physical therapy: a longitudinal study. *Archives of Physical Medicine and Rehabilitation* 95 (2):303–8.

Walton, D. M., Lefebvre, A., Reynolds, D., 2015. The Brief Illness Perceptions Questionnaire identifies 3 classes of people seeking rehabilitation for mechanical neck pain. *Manual Therapy* 20 (3):420–6.

Walton, D. M., Kwok, T. S., Mehta, S., et al., 2016. Cluster analysis of an International Pressure Pain Threshold database identifies 4 meaningful subgroups of adults with mechanical neck pain. *The Clinical Journal of Pain* 33 (5):422–8.

Wang, D., Pan, H., Zhu, H., et al., 2017. Upregulation of nuclear factor-κB and acid sensing ion channel 3 in dorsal root ganglion following application of nucleus pulposus onto the nerve root in rats. *Molecular Medicine Reports:* 16 (4): 4309–14.

3

A New Framework for Clinical Assessment of Musculoskeletal Pain

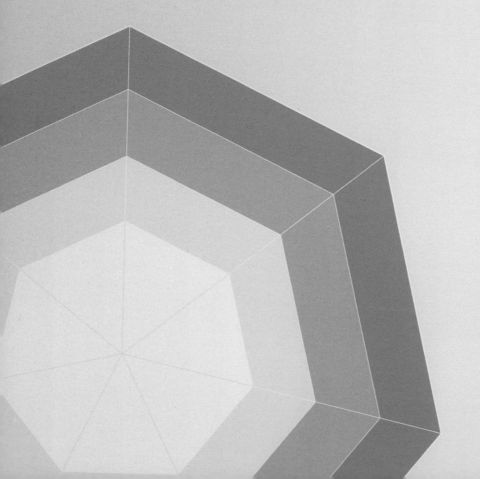

In this chapter we dive deeper into the two new frameworks that clinicians can use to facilitate the assessment and interpretation of complex pain or mobility problems. As mentioned in Chapter 2, we dedicate an entire section – and indeed the majority – of this book to the concept of assessment. We believe a sound assessment (and proper interpretation thereof) permits for a more confident prediction, and for subsequent treatment decisions to flow naturally and easily on a patient-by-patient basis. The complexity of the human condition, in particular a human that is also in pain or facing a threat to their sense of self, makes comprehensive assessment and evaluation difficult without a framework upon which to structure the process.

While we will not ignore the potential value of performing and interpreting the findings from a traditional biomechanical assessment, this section will not endorse a traditional biomechanical approach to assessment *in isolation*. Many luminaries of physical rehabilitation and medicine have come before us and provided frameworks that continue to be delivered in our entry-level classrooms and used in professional clinical practice today. These include, but are not limited to, Geoffrey Maitland, James Cyriax, Freddy Kaltenborn, Robin McKenzie, Gwendolen Jull, Shirley Sahrmann, and Brian Mulligan. Assessment through repeated movements, length-tension testing, or joint accessory glides, as described initially by leaders in the field, are common approaches used by non-medical and medical healthcare providers. While these approaches are probably a part of the broader picture of pain, in themselves they cannot identify the primary drivers of pain in isolation without considering the findings in the context of the broader picture of the person. As described previously, pain, like anger, fear, love, jealousy or hate, is complex and multifactorial, requiring simultaneous integration of information from multiple domains to offer even a glimpse of the 'actual' reality of the patient's experience. Psychologists and social workers, radiologists, anesthetists, occupational therapists, pharmacists and other professionals all conduct patient assessment from within their own disciplinary paradigms

to make diagnostic, prognostic and theranostic treatment decisions. While it can be a challenge to consider all of these sources of information at once, we believe the time for a new framework is now. A framework where all of the disparate data being collected are brought into a common paradigm where associations can be explored, common languages developed, and deeper learning across disciplines can occur.

It has become clearer that the individual experiences of pain and disability extend beyond the magnitude of damage to peripheral tissues and subsequent inflammation. Maladaptive or inaccurate beliefs, cognitions, or attributions about the pain appear to contribute at least as much to the experience of pain, or the reported severity thereof, as do tissue lesions (Vangronsveld et al., 2008; Khan et al., 2011). Emotional pathology related to distress or aversion seems to be maintained alongside pain in complex ways (Ravn et al., 2018; Ravn et al., 2019). Damage to peripheral nerves (neuropathic pain) (Sterling & Pedler, 2009) or changes to the pathways and chemical messengers in the central nervous system (central nociplastic change or *central sensitization*) (Woolf, 2011) appear common in some pain conditions and very likely contribute to the overall clinical picture. Information from the other senses (vision, touch, proprioception) seem to affect the experience of pain especially when the information being received is discordant with what is being perceived and reported by the person in pain (Field et al., 2008; Moseley, 2008). Socio-environmental (contextual) influences form a sort of over-arching layer within which all personal experiences occur and are given meaning. As such, the social determinants of pain are also, quite rightly, receiving increasing attention (McBeth & Jones, 2007; Carroll et al., 2011; Rudolph et al., 2011). Clinicians should consider the value of assessing the patient in pain from all of these perspectives as a critical step towards clinical decision-making beyond a simple 0-10 numeric rating scale. The question of *why did this patient rate that pain at that number?* is an important one in our minds that is not always appreciated in the clinic. Further, we recognize this is a daunting task without clear diagnostic options and a guiding framework for interpreting the findings.

Fortunately, we have been developing and refining such a framework over the past several years. This started as a tool for teaching both pre- and post-professional learners participating in classes and workshops for managing neck pain, but has been so well-received that it has formed the primary foundation for a new assessment paradigm. At the heart of the assessment framework are two key concepts: **the radar plot** and **triangulation**. Used together, these two concepts facilitate not only interpretation of otherwise complex presentations and potential interactions of multiple contributions to a patient's pain experience, but also facilitate the development of deep phenotyping and clinical pattern recognition. That latter function is particularly relevant to novice clinicians, as the past two decades' worth of research has revealed that one of the key differences between novice and expert clinicians is the ability of the latter to recognize patterns in clinical presentations that cannot be easily taught in classroom-based theoretical learning (May et al., 2008). By using the radar plot and triangulation concepts, novice clinicians can more accurately emulate the clinical pattern recognition skills of experts, and experts can explore complex pain presentations in even greater detail while keeping the messaging to their patients and other stakeholders relatively simple. These two concepts are explained here in greater detail, then expanded and reinforced throughout the subsequent chapters.

Why assess?

Hopefully we've managed to grab your attention on recognizing the value of sound assessment and evaluation of your patients in pain, and you're already starting to think beyond the traditional and sometimes mechanical approaches learned in health professional training programs. There is of course a larger issue here that we find is not always given due consideration: why

do we assess patients in the first place? On the surface this seems like a silly question with an obvious answer – *to identify the tissue at fault so that a targeted treatment plan can be made*. Indeed, that's one very logical answer, though as we've already described, in many pain conditions identifying a specific 'tissue at fault' is either difficult or impossible using mainstream, and often very expensive, clinical tools. We propose there are several reasons to conduct a sound patient assessment/evaluation beyond specific diagnoses, that will be discussed to help frame our subsequent sections.

Think about the last time you went to your personal family doctor with a feeling like something wasn't quite right in your own body. What were you hoping to get? Maybe a diagnostic label of your condition, which would help to answer the inevitable questions from concerned loved ones at home, friends, or colleagues at work? Perhaps you wanted to know what was causing it? Or you wanted to know how long you should expect it to take before you feel better, and if you or your doctor could/should be doing anything to help it improve more quickly? Maybe you needed some peace of mind that there wasn't anything sinister going on that could represent a serious threat to your health and well-being, or wanted to know if any additional tests were in order.

Your doctor, quite intuitively, would probably be thinking along similar lines but possibly for different reasons. Providers commonly require some kind of diagnostic code for practice and billing purposes, though realistically the diagnostic label itself is usually not critical to providing a treatment. Whether they call it by a mechanistic label: 'a *Streptococcus pneumoniae* infection of the right lower lobe' or give it the common diagnostic label of streptococcal pneumonia (ICD-10 code: J13), the treatment doesn't really change. They do of course want to prevent the death of patients in their charge. Accordingly, they will access their own archives of medical knowledge, expertise and experience to decide what, if any, treatment should be administered. They will consider if referral to another practitioner is required. And, in this case, the goal being prevention of mortality, they will choose a treatment that should hasten recovery. They'll also be thinking about public health issues and whether they need to recommend quarantine or hospitalization, whether they're confident in the diagnosis based on the information they have or if there is enough uncertainty that additional tests are required, and sometimes may explore other causal factors with you, such as your general physical health (past and current), the air quality in your home or workplace, stress, or exhaustion.

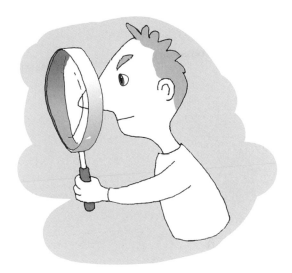

Here however we're going to go even deeper and break down the different functions of a sound assessment. For the purposes of creating a shared language, we will first define four different functions of clinical assessment, and the important properties of tools or techniques used for each function.

1. **Diagnosis/screening**. It's hard to argue against the value of diagnostic labels in today's culture. Whether it's considered from the context of the patient's desires and well-being, payors who require a diagnostic code, facilitating communication with other members of the healthcare team, or applying relevant clinical guidelines or algorithms, having a diagnostic label serves a value if it does not, in itself, always lead to a clear treatment pathway. In our experience, diagnosis tends to occur through either clinician intuition and pattern recognition considering all signs and symptoms, or through standardized, usually quantitative, clinical tests (blood tests, imaging, vitals, etc.). The use of the former is difficult to teach and even harder to study, though we know it exists as we've all had experiences with clinicians who just seem to be excellent diagnosticians without

requiring a lot of tests. When standardized tests are used, those with enough scientific evidence behind them will likely provide some statistical indication of just how confident you can be in making a diagnosis. There exists any number of fairly common statistics (e.g. sensitivity, specificity, negative and positive predictive value, negative and positive likelihood ratios, odds ratios, or relative risk) that you can find for many clinical diagnosis and screening tests, and when applied properly may help you decide whether you're 60% confident this patient has condition X or 90% confident. An example of this using a neuropathy screening tool is described later.

2. **Prognosis/theranosis: determining suitability for, or requirement of, your intervention.** Sound assessment should help you answer the question of whether this patient actually requires *any* intervention, and if so, whether the intervention you can offer is likely to be of value. For example, after making a mechanistic diagnosis of rhinovirus infection

(clinical diagnosis of a common cold), a doctor is unlikely to provide much intervention beyond a prescription for some rest and maybe some recommendations for symptom modification strategies, but is unlikely to order further tests. This is because they know two key pieces of information: first, that most common colds resolve spontaneously within about 7 to 10 days, meaning that the *prognosis* is good. Second, that there is little evidence that any kind of treatment will improve the rate of recovery from rhinovirus infection, meaning that the *theranosis* is poor.

Those two terms, prognosis and theranosis, should become part of your clinical lexicon. **Prognosis** refers to the expected outcome of a condition, usually in the absence of intervention (natural course) though sometimes intervention is considered in broad terms, like 'with surgery' or 'with physiotherapy' (clinical course). **Theranosis** refers to the likelihood that the patient's condition will improve with the introduction or application of a specific intervention or therapy. This information should be gleaned as part of your sound assessment strategy – what's the likelihood this person is going to get better (full-stop), and what's the likelihood that the interventions I can offer are going to affect that? We'll discuss prognosis issues further in Chapter 5.

3. **Determining where to direct your interventions.** Not everything has a tidy diagnostic label associated with it; things like 'chronic pain', 'non-specific low back pain', or 'headache' are really symptoms more than they are diagnoses. As a result, it's difficult to find intervention strategies or guidelines that can be confidently applied to the person sitting in front of you.

How, without a gold-standard, and biologically-based, diagnostic test (or tests), do we make sense of a practitioner's diagnosis? Should we value diagnostic signs (tests) more than the patient's personal reports and experience of their chronic pain, low back pain (LBP), or headache? Some rhetorical questions around the lack of diagnostics for, say, low back pain could be: 1) What is low back pain? 2) Is *it* 'nothing' since 'something' infrequently reveals itself on conventional imaging tests? 3) How do we measure *it*? So, rather than attempting to affix a distinct mechanism-based diagnostic label to a condition such as LBP, how about rethinking the value of a sound assessment used to triangulate any number of different components or domains of the patient's experience and the factors that are most likely driving their complaints?

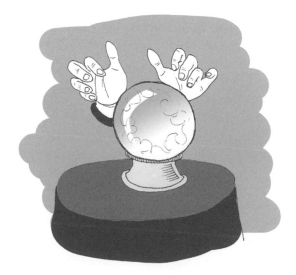

Moreover, in this way, you have a place from which to start a more informed treatment plan on a patient-by-patient basis. We get into this in far more detail in subsequent sections so will not dwell on it here, other than to say that assessment does not always lead to a diagnosis, but should lead to less uncertainty about where, how, when and to whom to direct your tailored treatments.

4. **Assessing any effect.** It is widely recognized through survey studies and anecdotal evidence that many clinicians across most health disciplines **do not** routinely capture any quantifiable metric of treatment effect or patient status. In response to the question of 'How do you know if your patient is getting better?', most will reply with something like 'I can see they're moving better' or 'they tell me they're feeling better'. This may be acceptable in more acute conditions: they were off for a couple of days, now they're back to work and all seems fine. Even here however, you're using work status as an outcome, and truth be told you don't *really* know if they've recovered or are working despite ongoing problems. However, in many chronic conditions this is even more problematic as there are many people who are 'working, despite being disabled', having found ways to push through a work day but are not in fact feeling very good about it.

In both acute and chronic pain conditions, we stress the value of becoming familiar with capturing some kind of *Patient-Reported Outcome* (PRO) on at least a semi-routine basis. A good PRO can provide a semi-quantifiable metric of the 'baseline' status of the patient, or where they started health-wise the first time they saw you. These can be useful prognostic tools as we'll discuss later and having this baseline data permits the valuable opportunity to re-administer the tool again later, after some reasonable time has passed, to see if (from the patient's perspective) things seem to be improving. We call these 'semi-quantifiable' in that they will provide a number, say out of 10 or out of 100, but they are not purely objective because they are, by definition, dependent on the patient to complete. This means they are susceptible to all of the biases related to self-report, including the degree to which the patient is paying attention, has understood the instructions and the questions (items) on the scale, has opinions on those items that make their reports meaningful, the degree to which they like you, may be trying to please you as their provider, other things going on in their lives, their mood, the importance of those items to that person, their literacy, and any number of other influences. However, accepting the inherent biases (and hoping that at least when measured serially within the same patient those biases are systematic rather than random) these really do give you a good sense of 'the view from in here'.

In today's thrust towards patient-centered care, the patient's perspective is (or at least should be) considered the closest to a 'gold standard' of the patient's health we have. PROs, we argue, should be useful to supplement the patient's narrative and your own clinical impressions, and together provide a richer picture of their actual health status. In summary, it doesn't *really* matter how well *you* think the patient is doing. If they don't think they're doing well, they're still going to experience (or at least perceive) impaired function and will likely continue to seek care, so it behooves you to collect some kind of metric of their condition beyond a 'How ya doing today?' informal question.

Hopefully that's enough to get you thinking about why we endorse a sound clinical assessment that goes beyond standardized or pre-defined questions and is conducted with deliberate thought, genuine curiosity, and consideration of the patient's well-being. In the next sections we will describe the two components of the APT framework that are intended to help you make sense of all the wonderful information you are (or will be) collecting.

The radar plot

A radar plot (introduced in Chapter 2, Fig. 2.2) is a valuable tool for creating and displaying profiles of a patient's presentation. It is a particularly valuable graphing tool when location on multiple domains are to be displayed on the same plot. Conceivably other types of plots (bar or line graphs) could accomplish the same thing, but the value of the radar plot is its ease of interpretation to even lay users (e.g. the general public). When used correctly, it forms a sort of compass that often points directly to the domain(s) of the pain experience that should be the primary (then secondary, tertiary, etc.) target(s) of intervention.

The sample radar plot displayed in Chapter 2 is one that we have used for our workshops on neck pain, but it holds relevance for pain in other regions of the body (i.e. low back, lower or upper extremities). In its current form it is a seven-point plot, with each point representing a different system or contributor to the experience of pain and disability that should be amenable to a different type of intervention. This latter point is of particular importance: it would be of little value to include domains in this plot that do not offer clear treatment guidance, and at the same time it is of little value to group too many domains together such that treatment decisions are unclear or ambiguous. The seven domains have been chosen with purpose based on several years of research and clinical experience, yet should remain fluid as new information emerges.

The domains themselves are not the critical point here, rather the concept of exploring pain from several domains and presenting them in such a way that providers and patients can understand them is the critical contribution. You may choose to evaluate different domains for your patient population – for example those working in concussion/mild traumatic brain injury, or post-surgical pain, or migraine headache may choose different domains, but the value is in the presentation and interpretation of data and the flexibility that this approach affords for allowing multiple (possibly interacting) pain drivers in the same patient.

As described in the philosophy section, the value of the radar plot approach is that we're moving away from the current trend of sub-grouping patients into tidy boxes. This leads to creation of a profile or *phenotype* with each point of the radar offering potential treatment options rather than a specific category with a limited set of treatment options. The current evidentiary base provides more qualitative than quantitative guidance for creating the plot (though the latter is quickly gaining steam). As of this writing then, the plot is developed through a mix of qualitative and quantitative means, but there is currently no mathematical algorithm for rating someone in the very low, low, moderate, high or very high categories (these are in fact intentionally described in qualitative terms given the current state of knowledge in many of the domains). With time, increased data, and increased accessibility to high-level machine-learning approaches, we anticipate that algorithmic creation of these profiles will become adequately valid and maybe even commonplace. However, for those who think better in mathematical terms, it is reasonable to consider the magnitude of contribution from each domain in terms of diagnostic/screening tools that usually provide things like sensitivity, specificity, likelihood ratios and posterior probabilities. So it should, in theory, be possible to consider the likelihood that one domain (e.g. peripheral neuropathy) is contributing to a patient's pain experience with a pre-test probability based on what you know of the patient to that point (e.g. peripheral symptom onset coincided with a mechanism of injury that could have caused damage to a peripheral nerve, complaints of symptoms affecting the distribution of a specific peripheral sensory innervation pattern, and complaints of paroxysmal symptoms like tingling, burning or pricking pain). Using these examples, a clinician may form a pre-test probability of a strong peripheral neuropathic driver being, let's say, 75% (which is probably somewhat conservative here). Then perhaps apply a tool of known diagnostic properties, such as the Self-report version of the Leeds Assessment of Neuropathic Signs and Symptoms (S-LANSS), and with a positive result (score >12), the post-test probability shifts to about 92% (assuming sensitivity (true positive) and specificity (true negative) of 0.80 for the S-LANSS (Bennett et al., 2005)). It's up to the clinician to decide whether 92% confidence translates to a higher or very high contribution to the patient's pain experience, a decision that seems straightforward on the surface until you stop to consider that there are simultaneously up to six other possible contributions, and the contributions from each are meant to be interpreted in more relative terms. If there are strong signs of both neuropathy *and* exaggerated negative cognitions for example, are these both very high contributors or is one very high and the other high? In practice these finer nuances may not be terribly important, both domains probably warrant intervention, but where to start is a decision that needs to be reached for each patient independently, which is why we're not jumping to the creation of mathematical algorithms.

Table 3.1 has been provided here to describe some potential tools, signs, symptoms or observations that may point towards or away from each of the seven key domains. These will be described in greater detail in the following sections. Looking at it, one reasonable question (and one we've been asked countless times) is: just how many tools do you use with these patients anyway? Fortunately, the answer is not as many as you may think, and in fact, thinking in terms of a radar

plot and profile will very likely take no longer than your current routine of clinical evaluation – it may even be shorter.

We will describe tools in the coming sections that provide rich information for estimating patient locations on several domains in a single scale or test. There are many tests for which a positive finding leads to greater strength in one domain while reducing the likelihood of a problem in another. Take active cervical range of motion for example: reduced range of motion in multiple planes or with pain in an inconsistent (non-mechanical) pattern may strengthen your confidence in a more central nociplastic component while simultaneously reducing the likelihood of a strong mechanical (physiological) nociceptive component. The reciprocal of that would also be true: a pattern of restriction and/or pain that is consistent and congruent with what would be expected from a particular tissue lesion (e.g. a clear 'facet compression' pattern) strengthens the likelihood of contribution from physiological peripheral nociceptive input while reducing the likelihood of strong contribution from central mechanisms.

Another strategy we endorse in this book is the use of a 'go-to' toolbox, that is a set of PROs that all patients complete when they come for their first visit, before you even lay a hand or eyes upon them. This toolbox should be one that includes *at most* three to four scales of known measurement properties that also tap into several of the radar plot domains. None of them may be enough on its own to offer 'high' or 'very high' confidence of any domain, but together they may be enough to rule out some domains allowing you to focus your subsequent assessment on those that are most likely to be strong contributors. The combination of your go-to toolbox before seeing the patient (and proper interpretation thereof, a discussion yet to come), well-conceived and intentional questions during the patient history and interview,

Table 3.1 Indicators for the seven radar plot domains

Nociceptive (mechanical, chemical, thermal)	Peripheral neuropathic	Central neurogenic	Sensorimotor dysintegration	Cognitive	Affective/emotional	Social/environmental
Adaptive, orthodromic, protective May still exhibit signs of peripheral sensitization	Pathological, peripheral nerve injury, orthodromic and antidromic	Changes in the CNS that lead to an environment of nociceptive facilitation	Changes in the CNS that lead to discordant sensory and motor integration	Thoughts, beliefs, values or perceptions that affect interpretation and suffering	Diagnosable or definable clinical or subclinical psychopathology	Contextual factors that interact with biological and psychological factors to influence interpretation, reporting, and other behaviors
• 'Mechanical' pattern of reproduction – predictable and consistent • Makes anatomical sense • Local hyperalgesia • Responsive to appropriate OTC medication (e.g. NSAIDs) • Predictable diurnal patterns	• History (obvious or likely) of nerve trauma • Non-mechanical patterns, spontaneous pain localized to innervation territory of lesioned nerve • Sensory loss: hypoesthesia, hypoalgesia • Sensory gain: allodynia, hyperalgesia • Dysesthesias: electric, shocking, burning, cold, heavy, itching, crawling • Screening tools: S-LANSS (≥ 12/24), DN4 (≥4/10) or PainDETECT (≥19/38) • Localized wind-up pain	• Longer-term duration of symptoms • Non-mechanical patterns of symptom reproduction • Diagnostic findings clear or equivocal • Widespread sensory hyperalgesia • Dysfunctional conditioned pain modulation • Central Sensitivity Index (≥40/100) • Usually associated with other symptoms inc. digestive, sleep, cognitive, sensory or motor interference	• Poor laterality recognition • Increased joint position sense error • Increased postural sway • Impaired two-point discrimination • Abnormal oculomotor/righting reflexes • Increased protective muscle tone (guarding in response to unknown limb or joint position) • Clinical or subclinical motor ataxia (clumsiness, difficulty mastering exercise) • Problems with reading, swallowing, or voice projection (esp. in neck pain)	• Catastrophic beliefs (PCS >20) • Fear of movement/injury (FABQ, TSK) • Sense of victimization (IEQ) • Low self-efficacy beliefs (PSEQ) • Poor expectations of recovery (BIPQ) • Generalized trauma-related distress (TIDS) • Any number of other cognitive tools	• Major/minor depressive disorder (PHQ-9 or HADS) • Generalized anxiety disorder (HADS, DASS) • Post-traumatic stress disorder (PCL, PDS, IES) • Somatoform disorder • Borderline personality disorder, narcissism • Social phobias • Obsessive compulsive disorder	• Spousal responses • Job satisfaction • Job laterality • Unpaid/gendered roles • Compensation • Litigation • Access to care • Cultural norms • Ethnic norms • Previous life experiences

CNS, Central nervous system; OTC, over the counter.
Tool abbreviations: BIPQ, Brief Illness Perceptions Questionnaire; DASS, Depression, Anxiety, and Stress Scale; DN4, Douleur Neuropathique 4; FABQ, Fear-Avoidance Beliefs Questionnaire; HADS, Hospital Anxiety and Depression Scale; IEQ, Injustice Experience Questionnaire; IES, Impact of Event Scale; PCL, PTSD Checklist; PCS, Pain Catastrophizing Scale; PDS, PTSD Diagnosis Scale; PHQ9, Patient Health Questionnaire 9; PSEQ, Pain Self-Efficacy Questionnaire; S-LANSS, Self-report version of the Leeds Assessment of Neuropathic Signs and Symptoms; TIDS, Traumatic Injuries Distress Scale; TSK,Tampa Scale for Kinesiophobia.

and a few robust clinical tests will probably provide more than enough data once you digest it to construct a very useful patient profile. In fact we believe that the patient history and interview is the most critical step of the entire interaction: if you ask the right questions and listen well enough, the patient will probably tell you what's wrong and what you need to do about it – you just need to be prepared to hear it.

We will encourage you to become familiar with several tools and scales, both patient-reported and clinician-administered, but it may be rare that you need to use more than the three or four in your go-to toolbox. However, the value of being familiar with the individual items, including the phrases or terms used in each, will better prepare you to pick up subtle clues in your patients' stories. For example, when a patient begins describing feelings of helplessness or an inability to think of anything other than the pain, this may clue you in to catastrophic beliefs based on your knowledge of the questions and subdomains of the widely used Pain Catastrophizing Scale (PCS). It would then be up to you as the clinician to decide whether you need to have the patient formally complete a PCS in order to better quantify these cognitions and have a score on the chart, perhaps to use for communication with other providers, or as a baseline to track change. But the patient's story may be enough to allow you to construct a profile if you're already familiar with the questions asked on those scales. In this way, the approach we're endorsing is meant to respect both the best available evidence, your own experience, intuition or heuristics as a clinician, and of course the patient's context, values and beliefs. This is the essence of true evidence-informed patient-centered care, which should be the goal of every clinician.

There is an important social perspective on PROs however that we wish to briefly address, and that is the often paternalistic, potentially even (unintentionally) harmful impacts on the patient of assigning ranks, scores, or labels as a result of responses on a scale. While most are designed with a spirit of 'there is no right answer here, we're only collecting your personal beliefs', those scales that then offer diagnostic groupings on the basis of those 'personal beliefs' do, in many ways, suggest there are indeed right and wrong answers. This is an often unrecognized and, we believe, underappreciated and underexplored effect of many PROs *especially* those that offer thresholds (e.g. mildly, moderately, or severely disabled). This issue has yet to be reconciled in healthcare, especially by advocates of strong clinical measurement (ourselves included), though as you will read throughout this book, this is one of the strong drivers behind our messaging that the summed scores on such tools are *less* useful for clinical decision-making than are the patterns of responses to individual items. When used in this way (exploring the actual responses, not just the sum of scores) not only does a well-constructed PRO offer plenty of information for triangulation, but should also open valuable conversation paths based on those items that patients strongly endorse.

Triangulation

Triangulation is the second new concept we want clinicians to consider during patient interactions and should be used alongside phenotyping to construct a sound radar plot. In fact, the use of the terms 'radar' and 'triangulation' are quite intentional, as triangulation is a term borrowed from positioning techniques first used by radar technicians in World War II. While new radar technologies no longer require triangulation to pinpoint the location of targets, original radar techniques required information from more than one receiver dish to accurately locate an object's location. Newer technologies in other fields continue to use this concept, such as the way in which smartphone maps can pinpoint your location to within meters (or less) even when inside a building. Imagine the phone in your pocket is visible (connected) to a mobile phone/

cellular transmission tower with an effective radius of 1+ km and, based on the strength of the signal, the software doing the locating knows you are 1 km from that tower. Of course, that could be any point on a circle with a 1 km radius (2km diameter), which is not very precise. But then imagine your phone is also visible to another cell tower with a similar 1+ km effective radius. Software processing can now narrow your location to the overlap between the 1 km radius of the first tower and the 1.75km radius of the second, which is two possible points. If a third, less power-ful tower can also see your device right at the edge of its range (500 m), there is only one possible point of overlap between the 1 km, 1.75 km and 500 m radii of the three towers where you could be located (Fig. 3.1). In this way, the mapping software can pinpoint your location with high accuracy by using and interpreting these three sources of information together. To put it

another way, if it walks like a duck, looks like a duck, and quacks like a duck (three independent sources of information), you can be fairly confident that you are looking at a duck.

The APT framework encourages the use of trian-gulation when constructing a patient profile. In this context we refer to triangulating a patient's position on each of the seven domains of the radar plot, espe-cially for something as invisible and personal as pain or disability. Here the triangulation occurs when the results from at least three *different sources of infor-mation* all point towards the same domain of the radar plot. This could be any combination of posi-tive findings on assessment techniques that target that domain, and negative findings on techniques that target alternative domains. We especially value three different tests that 'tap' the domain from

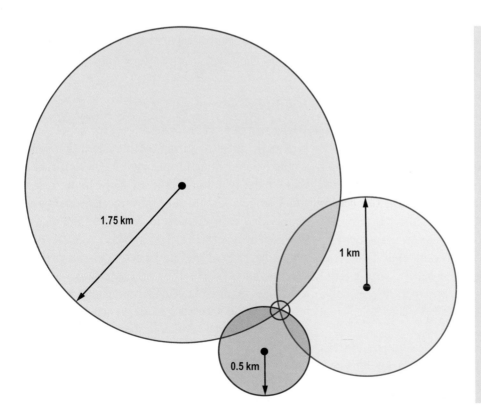

Figure 3.1
A graphical depiction of the concept of triangula-tion. If the distance from a center (e.g. a cell phone tower) is known to be 1 km, the object (e.g. a phone) can be anywhere within that 1 km radius. When a second tower, 1.75 km away is also able to 'see' the device, there are two possible points that those two radii overlap at which the device can be located. If a third tower, in this example a less powerful one, can see the device 500m away, there is only one possible location that all three radii overlap where the device could be located (circled in red).

different directions. So, while three different self-report tools might help you get there, we'd be more excited by convergent findings from a self-report tool, a clinical test, and maybe something from the patient's history or a result from diagnostic imaging. When all three of these things point towards the same position on a domain (e.g. low, moderate, high or very high), we would say that you have triangulated that patient's position on that domain. Of course, as mentioned in the previous section, it would be ideal if every clinical assessment outcome also had an associated positive or negative likelihood ratio, such that a clinician could calculate an actual *post-test probability* that dysfunction in a particular domain is driving or contributing to that patient's clinical condition. Alas, whilst evidence is growing, there are still relatively few clinical techniques for which such information is available. However, the concept of triangulation (three independent sources of evidence for each domain) should be more than adequate to determine the strength of

the contribution from that domain. A mathematical example of this is shown in Table 3.2.

These concepts (radar plot, phenotyping, triangulation) may at first seem overwhelming and it's not surprising if you are feeling a tad confused at this stage. These terms are not currently common in health professional training programs, though anecdote tells us they are starting to creep up here and there. As with any new approach to clinical practice, while clumsy and cumbersome at first, it will get easier with time and practice. Clinicians with a very quantitative bent to their practice may feel somewhat disappointed that creating a good patient profile is not a purely mathematical endeavor, though the math is admittedly beginning to improve. Proficiency in these approaches, and dare we say true proficiency as a clinician, requires a blend of both instrumental skills in selecting and applying the right tests, and interpersonal skills in asking good questions, connecting on a deeper level,

Table 3.2 Sample triangulation using likelihood ratios				
Assumptions for this example:				
Pre-test probability that condition exists (odds) 50% (1:2)				
	Discriminative validity	Likelihood ratios (LR)	Post-test probability all tests positive	Post-test probability all tests negative
Clinical test 1	Sn 0.80, Sp 0.80	+LR 4.00, −LR 0.25	67% (2:1)	11% (1:8)
Clinical test 2	Sn 0.75, Sp 0.75	+LR 3.00, −LR 0.33	86% (6:1)	4% (1:25)
Clinical test 3	Sn 0.66, Sp 0.67	+LR 2.00, −LR 0.51	92% (12:1)	2% (1:50)

With three tests, each of modest to low discriminative validity, but each positive, the likelihood that a condition exists (or that a particular mechanism on the radar plot is important) goes from 50% to 92%, suggesting that domain should be in the high to very high range of the plot. If all three tests are negative, the likelihood a domain is a strong driver goes from 50% to 2%, moving that domain to low or very low. Both calculations are conducted accepting some likely inflation due to ignoring the prior odds fallacy. (Reproduced with permission from Walton, D.M., Elliott, J.M., 2018. A new clinical model for facilitating the development of pattern recognition skills in clinical pain assessment. *Musculoskeletal Science and Practice* 36:17–24.)

Chapter 3

and listening actively to pick up clues from patient narratives as they come up.

The following chapters will describe patient-level variables that should be considered when interpreting any set of clinical tests. Then we describe the 'go-to' toolbox with suggestions of PROs that clinicians who are considering use of the radar plot and triangulation concepts can adopt into their practice, though they are just that: suggestions. Subsequent chapters will then explore each of the seven domains in a more targeted fashion describing the proposed mechanisms of each as a driver of the pain experience, empirically derived clinical tools where available, and other clues or sources of information from patient narratives that can be used in place of, or to complement, standardized tools. In all cases we have intentionally discussed tools, especially the self-report tools, that are freely available in the public domain or can at least be used by clinicians for free with permission of the creator. Every one of the tools we describe can be found with a simple Google search. In some cases, there may be tools that are protected under copyright and patent law that have better discriminative properties than free ones but require payment to legally use. In those cases, we will give a nod to their existence in case readers should wish to explore them further, but they will not be a focus of our discussion. As with anything, readers are encouraged to first explore any tool they are considering using to ensure that the copyright holder has made it freely available.

References

Bennett, M. I., Smith, B. H., Torrance, N., et al., 2005. The S-LANSS score for identifying pain of predominantly neuropathic origin: validation for use in clinical and postal research. *The Journal of Pain : Official Journal of the American Pain Society* 6 (3):149–58.

Carroll, L. J., Connelly, L. B., Spearing, N. M., et al., 2011. Complexities in understanding the role of compensation-related factors on recovery from whiplash-associated disorders: discussion paper 2. *Spine* 36 (25 Suppl):S316–21.

Field, S., Treleaven, J., Jull, G., 2008. Standing balance: a comparison between idiopathic and whiplash-induced neck pain. *Manual Therapy* 13 (3):183–91.

Khan, R. S., Ahmed, K., Blakeway E., et al., 2011. Catastrophizing: a predictive factor for postoperative pain. *American Journal of Surgery* 201 (1):122–31.

May, S., Greasely, A., Reeve, S., et al., 2008. Expert therapists use specific clinical reasoning processes in the assessment and management of patients with shoulder pain: a qualitative study. *The Australian Journal of Physiotherapy* 54 (4):261–6.

McBeth, J., Jones, K., 2007. Epidemiology of chronic musculoskeletal pain. *Best Practice & Research. Clinical Rheumatology* 21 (3):403–25.

Moseley, G. L., 2008. I can't find it! Distorted body image and tactile dysfunction in patients with chronic back pain. *Pain* 140 (1):239–43.

Ravn, S. L., Hartvigsen, J., Hansen, M., et al., 2018. Do post-traumatic pain and post-traumatic stress symptomatology mutually maintain each other? A systematic review of cross-lagged studies. *Pain* 159 (11): 2159–69.

Ravn, S. L., Karstoft, K. I., Sterling, M., et al., 2019. Trajectories of posttraumatic stress symptoms after whiplash: A prospective cohort study. *European Journal of Pain* 23 (3):515–25.

Rudolph, K. D., Troop-Gordon, W., Granger, D. A., 2011. Individual differences in biological stress responses moderate the contribution of early peer victimization to subsequent depressive symptoms. *Psychopharmacology* (Berl) 214 (1):209–19.

Sterling, M., Pedler, A., 2009. A neuropathic pain component is common in acute whiplash and associated with a more complex clinical presentation. *Manual Therapy* 14 (2):173–9.

Vangronsveld, K. L., Peters, M., Goossens, M., et al., 2008. The influence of fear of movement and pain catastrophizing on daily pain and disability in individuals with acute whiplash injury: a daily diary study. *Pain* 139 (2):449–57.

Woolf, C. J., 2011. Central sensitization: implications for the diagnosis and treatment of pain. *Pain* 152 (3 Suppl):S2-15.

4

Classifications of Patients that Matter when Interpreting Pain

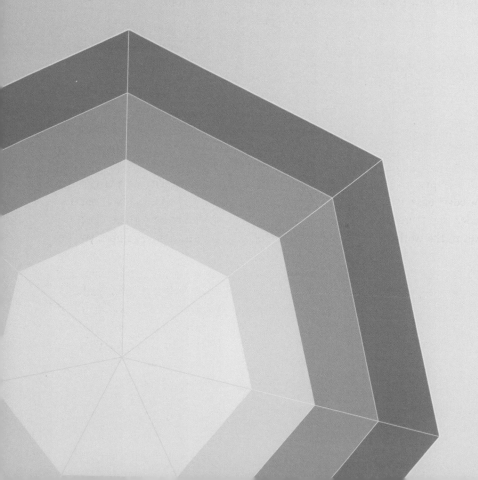

Before getting into the *go-to toolbox*, and the specific domains and details of what questions, scales and tools to use when and for what purpose, it is worth a brief discussion of some key considerations that may influence the tools you select and how you interpret their results. We have encouraged a move away from unique empirically derived subgroups or classifications towards multidimensional profiling (*phenotyping*) that simultaneously considers several distinct domains. This is mostly borne out of recognition that human beings rarely fit nicely into unique clinical categories, and that the categories have rarely stood up to repeated testing by independent groups. Some exceptions exist, such as Ritchie's prognostic algorithm for whiplash (Kelly et al., 2017) and Hill's algorithms using the STarT Back tool in low back pain (Hill et al., 2010), but those are currently rare.

However, there are very likely important patient-level characteristics that should be considered as you work towards creating a profile of a patient with pain. In simple terms, these characteristics include, but are not limited to, sex, duration of symptoms, mechanism of onset, and comorbidities. In the interest of optimizing translatability for clinicians (and other stakeholders – the patient included) we are again keeping the gradations of these different categories fairly simple. So, we will consider sex from a dichotomous (biological) male or female perspective, rather than say, the 71 different sex and gender options currently available on Facebook for user profiles.[1] Not surprisingly the scientific knowledge base is only recently paying attention to the idea that there are at least two different biological sexes in the world, and is not nearly precise enough to interpret pain evaluation from 71 different perspectives. Understanding the differences between biological *sex* and culturally constructed *gender* can be difficult, but it is important to realize that the characteristics of both sex and gender can affect pain perception and expressions. So, we'll keep it simple for now, at least to the extent that 'simple' is even possible in this field.

In broad strokes then, here are some important patient characteristics or classifications (if you prefer that term) that you should consider.

Sex: male or female

We put this consideration first as it's likely the easiest one to figure out (though not always obvious, remember those 71 Facebook options). The sex of your patient should influence how you interpret their responses and scores on a standardized tool, or performance on a standardized test, though we urge caution in making assumptions about mechanisms and are in no way endorsing 'sexist' interpretations of medical information. At the same time however, we believe that medicine should no longer remain what some have called 'gender blind'. Perhaps this isn't terribly profound, but men and women *are* different and very likely have different life experiences, values, expectations, and responses to intervention. For example, women outnumber men in most chronic pain populations meaning that when attempting to establish pre- and post-test probabilities for risk or prognosis, women most likely start at higher risk than men. This isn't a strong effect, it appears to be about a 1.5-fold increase on average at least in traumatic neck pain (Walton et al., 2013) but it's fairly consistent and not something to ignore. Notably, keep in mind that cause-and-effect has yet to be established: does being female *cause* chronic pain? Or are there other differences (confounders) that make women more likely to experience (or at least report experiencing) more intense or more frequent pain? That is a larger discussion for another time. However, the fact that differences appear to exist should have some effect on interpretation of clinical tests. If, for example, you do choose to use risk categories for estimating likelihood of recovery/developing chronic pain after traumatic neck or low back pain, you will find empirical evidence that tells you 25–35% of the entire population of people with acute injuries are likely low risk, 15–20% are likely high risk, and the remaining 45–60% are unclear risk. However, those numbers probably shake out slightly differently between the sexes.

[1] https://www.telegraph.co.uk/technology/facebook/10930654/Facebooks-71-gender-options-come-to-UK-users.html.

So, for women the ratios may be more like: low risk, 20–30%; high risk, 20–25%; unclear risk, 50–55% (Fig. 4.1A). While for men those may be: low risk, 30–40%; high risk, 10–15%; unclear risk, 45–60% (Fig. 4.1B). These differences may seem subtle but as evidence accrues, knowing the pre-test probabilities (ratios) is important, as that will permit calculation of an actual post-test probability on a patient-by-patient basis.

There are other important considerations for interpretation of standardized self-report or clinical (observational) tools for which sex of the patient should be considered. There is *almost* universal evidence to suggest that, on average, for a given stimulus intensity, women will rate the pain intensity higher than men (Bartley & Fillingim, 2013). Similarly, for pain thresholds, women will usually stop the test and report pain at a lower threshold than men (Walton et al., 2011). We and others have found this relationship many times across several different testing methods, so it's adequately consistent to say a difference exists on average. That is, of course, not to say that all women

will have lower pain thresholds and rate higher pain than some men, but when averaged across entire samples or populations, this seems to be most often the case. Causal mechanisms are no doubt complex and very likely include biological, psychological and social influences on how stimuli are processed, perceived, and reported that is only just recently receiving the attention it deserves. Alarmingly, and the reason we believe the conversation is worth having, is that considerable evidence exists to indicate that women are also less likely to receive adequate management of their pain than are their male counterparts (Hoffmann & Tarzian, 2001; Chen et al., 2008).

Beyond gender equity in pain management, the consistent findings of differences in pain ratings between the sexes should also influence interpretations of clinical scales. Take for example the consistent finding that high pain intensity shortly after a motor vehicle collision (MVC) is a consistent risk factor for chronic pain, as we and others have found many times (Walton et al., 2013). In our 2010 (updated in 2013) meta-analysis of risk factors for chronic whiplash, we found a cut-score of 5.5/10 as indicating high risk. In other words, those who rate 6/10 or higher on their intake pain intensity are more likely to earn membership to the high-risk group than are those who rate 5 or lower. Here again, this has yet to be explored separately for males and females, but if we assume the trends we've just presented hold true, then that 5.5/10 number should probably be something more like 4.5/10 for males (so 5 or higher) and 6.5/10 for females (7 or higher). That is, since men tend to rate their pain *on average* lower than women, those risk categories should probably be shifted accordingly. Casting a social justice lens towards this consideration should however reveal the potential for such an approach to contribute to gender-based health inequities (that is, the practice of setting the bar higher for females than for males when defining risk, and by extension, deciding who should receive more care). As of this writing

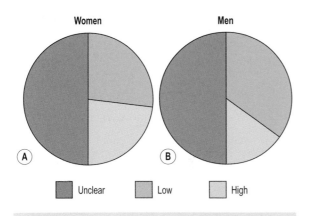

Figure 4.1
Estimating likelihood of recovery or for developing chronic pain after traumatic neck or low back pain in (**A**) women: low risk, 20–30%; high risk, 20–25%; unclear risk, 50–55%; and (**B**) men: low risk, 30–40%; high risk, 10–15%; unclear risk, 45–60%.

(2019), there is no simple way to reconcile this, and the world seems to be only recently coming to terms with the concept that females are not simply scaled down versions of males (an old medical and research adage, if largely unspoken). Our approach will be to endorse acknowledging and respecting that pain experience and reports thereof will likely be different, on average, between men and women, but that access to and the provision of care should remain equal.

A final consideration is that males and females very likely respond to items on standardized tests through different contextual lenses. Granted, when higher-level analyses of many common tools have been conducted, sex is rarely an important modifier of response. However, traditionally scale development has largely occurred through generation of items that, while often unspoken, most commonly apply to the average Caucasian male. Population-level data indicate that men and women often differ in many potentially important ways in terms of requirements for driving, working outside of the home, lifting, running, and so on. This is even more pronounced across different global cultures. So again, we must consider the effect of sex (and the cultural context of how one might respond to what is being asked) on responses to common tools. Another consideration is, for example, regardless of sex do people who do NOT drive (opting for public transport), or do NOT work tend to skip those questions? If they do answer them, how and why do they answer them since none of the response options really pertain to them? In these cases, you may decide that generic scales that include fewer specific activities are more appropriate for your patient population (explored further in the next chapters).

Where differences have been supported by evidence, we will point them out in the next chapters. Since sex- and gender-based analyses have traditionally been rare in pain research, this is more of a consideration than a hard and fast rule for most tools. But

reason for optimism does exist, in that as of January 2016 most major national health research funders, including the National Institutes of Health (the primary federal funding source of research in the United States) and the Canadian Institutes of Health Research (primary funder in Canada) established policies requiring all researchers to consider sex and gender in clinical and preclinical research.

Duration: acute or chronic

Considering the length of time your patient has lived with their current pain experience should influence both your choice of tools and your interpretation thereof. For the purposes of this consideration (and to continue to keep things as simple as possible), we'll consider 'acute' to be up to 3 to 6 weeks from onset, 'chronic' anything lasting 3 months or longer, and the 3 weeks to 3 months period a bit of a *gray zone*. You may recall that *gray zone* has often been labelled the 'subacute' phase, but the 'subacute' phase has rarely been the subject of targeted study, so the label is of questionable clinical utility. For those patients navigating the in-between gray zone of duration, let common sense prevail.

The biggest issue to consider here is validity of PROs, or the degree to which the response (or responses) you get to a question (or scale) will in fact be reflective of the construct you're trying to measure. From a purely research standpoint, many scales currently being used in practice have yet to undergo appropriate scrutiny for different symptom durations. This is especially true for many of the cognitive scales currently in use in chronic pain settings that clinicians and researchers have tried to shoehorn into the acute phase. These include the Pain Catastrophizing Scale, the Tampa Scale for Kinesiophobia, and the Fear-Avoidance Beliefs Questionnaire. Each have demonstrated adequate evidence of validity for use in chronic pain populations, but for the most part, and despite their increased use, their properties for use in the acute phase are far less clear.

Chapter 4

You need not be an expert in measurement properties to figure out what tools are appropriate for acute populations and what ones are not. One of the easiest things you can do is read and understand the actual scale yourself (an activity that we've learned relatively few clinicians undertake). Does it start by asking patients to consider their pain or function over the past 2 or 3 hours? Days? Weeks? If so, clearly the scale is not appropriate for anyone who has experienced the condition for less than that time, and only barely appropriate for those who have experienced it for exactly 2 or 3 weeks since things have likely been quite labile over that period. Even for those scales that don't provide a time window, reviewing the items and response options is also important. Do the items (the questions being asked) require the respondent to have lived with the condition for long enough to be able to form an opinion on them? If so, how long would that take? An hour? A day? A week? A month? And then look at the response options: if the responses are frequency based ('never' to 'every day'), how many days would it take for people to be able to answer 'every day'? The nature of *most* region-specific disability scales (such as the Neck Disability Index (NDI) or Oswestry Disability Index (ODI)) require people to have lived with the condition for at least a few days, and likely a week or longer to really form opinions on things like recreational activities, sleep, or work interference. So, consider this when choosing a scale.

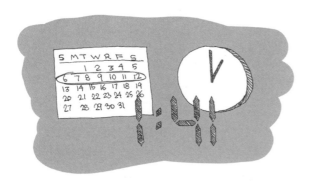

Then there are tools that are intended specifically for people with acute problems. Examples would be the STarT Back tool or the Orebro Musculoskeletal Pain Questionnaire as prognostic tools for acute low back pain. They lose their value as the condition becomes chronic, since the idea of prognostic subgrouping is no longer valuable; clearly the prognosis is poor if the person already has chronic pain. Similarly, post-traumatic distress is becoming a popular construct to measure (or at least consider) when working with patients exposed to trauma, but here again there are some tools that only hold meaning in the acute post-traumatic stage (e.g. the Acute Stress Reactions Questionnaire). Since the diagnosis of post-traumatic stress disorder (PTSD) can only be made after symptoms have been present for at least a month, such screening tools as the PTSD Diagnostic Scale (PDS; Foa et al., 1997), PTSD Checklist (PCL; Weathers et al., 1993) or Impact of Events Scale (IES; Horowitz et al., 1979) are only relevant for longer term conditions.

One final, but critical, consideration in this duration discussion is the purpose for which the assessment is being conducted. In the APT philosophy, these are different depending on whether the condition is in the acute or chronic stage. For those in the acute stage of pain, the focus of assessment should be **prognosis,** that is, estimating the likely outcome if no treatment is offered and delivered. Where the prognosis is poor (e.g. the person is unlikely to satisfactorily improve without treatment), the assessment then switches to a focus on identifying those risk factors that are modifiable, and thus amenable to intervention. Where the prognosis is favorable (e.g. the patient is likely to recover well), the strategy is to let nature take its course, avoid over-treatment and reduce the risk of *iatrogenic disability.* Once the condition has transitioned into the chronic stage (or more accurately, if the condition has failed to transition to recovery) then prognosis becomes less meaningful. Here the focus changes to **theranosis**, wherein you are attempting to estimate the likelihood that a patient's condition will respond to a treatment and how big an effect can be expected. Creating a profile (phenotype) of your patient with the radar plot would be of great value in this chronic group, permitting the identification and visual display of the modifiable domains requiring the most attention.

While sex may be the *easiest* patient characteristic to decipher, the difference between acute and chronic conditions is likely the *most important* consideration when choosing the most appropriate questions, scales or tests for your patient and how you interpret those. This way the clinical encounter is meaningful, and you gain rich information without wasting your or your patient's time on irrelevant and isolated measures.

Mechanism of onset: traumatic or insidious

Knowing whether the onset of the patient's condition was the result of a trauma (i.e. they can clearly trace the onset back to a specific event) or more insidious (i.e. developed or worsened over time without an obvious inciting event) is an important piece of information when choosing questions, scales, and tests. While this may seem elementary, unless you have some advance knowledge of the patient's condition, you may not know the mechanism of onset until you actually start talking with the patient. So, you may need to be adaptable and choose your 'go-to' tools (Chapter 5) in such a way that they are not specific to only one type of onset. This is an important piece of information as mechanistic differences between people with traumatic and non-traumatic onset of pain seem to exist. This is arguably truer in neck pain than most other body regions, but the consideration holds relevance across regions.

Keeping with the neck pain example, it's hard to get your neck 'whipped' without at least a bit of a head jiggle. That soft jelly-like structure inside the skull (the brain) and the traction-averse spinal cord are at greater risk of some degree of damage that could manifest as motor incoordination, concussion or concussion-like symptoms as a result. To wit, many in the field are now wondering if whiplash and concussion are in fact two distinct entities or would be better conceptualized as two different points along the same continuum of head-neck trauma. The overlap in mechanism of injury, symptoms, and recovery are strikingly similar between the two so this current line of thinking may not be far off the mark. Recognizing the potential for some degree of closed head injury or other neurological-type involvement that is more likely following a traumatic onset than an insidious or degenerative one, should influence your choice of tools, your interpretation of the patient's response(s) or performance on them, and of course your treatment decisions.

More generally, any pain resulting from trauma is far more likely to be associated with distress or anxiety-related problems than is pain from a more gradual, non-traumatic, onset. PTSD is becoming increasingly recognized, or at least increasingly explored, in traumatic pain and early evidence suggests it may be related to recovery in slightly strange ways (see Chapter 11 on emotional drivers for more). We, and others, have also found that people who identify trauma as their mechanism of onset (e.g. motor vehicle collision, slips and falls, workplace injuries, sporting injuries, assault) also tend to report higher levels of pain catastrophizing (Walton et al., 2012), lower pain thresholds to mechanical or thermal stimuli (Scott et al., 2005), and more signs of disordered central nociceptive transmission (Elliott et al., 2014) than do their non-traumatic counterparts. All this is to say that when you identify trauma as a mechanism of onset for your patient's pain, you should be thinking about a slightly different set of tools, change your expectations for what a 'normal' response will be, be prepared to pick up signs more indicative of a strong emotional driver, and set slightly different thresholds of response or performance than those patients with insidious-onset problems. Where these are obvious in the chapters on different drivers, we will point them out.

Comorbidities

No simple dichotomy on this one, but knowing your patient's current and past medical history is going to be an important influence on how you interpret the results of your different tools, if not how you select them in the first place. Some of these considerations are simple; if your patient suffered a large shin contusion as a result of the motor vehicle crash that also caused neck pain, then chances are the results of pressure pain detection threshold testing over the tibialis anterior (as we will discuss in the section on nociceptive vs. central drivers) will not be appropriate or reasonably interpretable. But more nuanced are those increasingly common *chronic* comorbidities that may influence the way a patient responds to common tools and clinical tests. One example of this would be screening tools for anxiety disorders that are very likely confounded by the presence of musculoskeletal pain. For example, the Hospital Anxiety and Depression Scale (HADS) includes an item asking people to rate their agreement with the statement 'I can sit at ease and feel relaxed'. This is meant to tap the construct of anxiety, but clearly someone with disabling neck or back pain will have an awfully hard time sitting at ease and feeling relaxed, regardless of how anxious they feel. Pre-existing psychopathology (e.g. depression, anxiety, substance use disorder) will likely have unexpected effects on responses to self-report questionnaires: does a high score on a Pain Catastrophizing Scale in fact mean that the person is misunderstanding their pain, or could it be an effect of an underlying depressive disorder? It is worth knowing (or even exploring) as the interventions based on such interpretations will be very different. Even on clinical tests, differences may manifest: it is not uncommon for depression to be associated with

lower pain thresholds and widespread bodily pain even in those who do not also endorse a chronic pain disorder. Sleep disorders such as insomnia have also been shown to reduce pain threshold, adversely affect emotions and impair higher-level cognitive processes (Schuh-Hofer et al., 2013).

Chronic systemic diseases, or even temporary health conditions, will almost certainly influence a patient's response to a scale or question or their performance on a test, dependent on the condition. This is an area in which research falls woefully short. While many studies will exclude participants with psychopathology, almost all will also have excluded those with cancer, major organ disease, or neurological conditions (unless the nature of the study was particularly targeting that condition). Even pregnant or post-partum women have often been excluded from test design studies, prognostic research, and clinical intervention trials. The truth is, most of the empirical knowledge we hold regarding how best to assess, predict and treat pain has come from studies with very 'clean' patient samples who may not represent the messy reality of clinical practice. This is where the concepts of the radar plot and triangulation become even more critical. You may find yourself relying more on experience and intuition in patients with multimorbidity. But you may also find it a good strategy to combine your experience and intuition with multiple sources of information from different angles to create a profile of the patient's pain condition. The latter strategy being one that will prevent you from prematurely acting on a single piece of information without adequately considering the full picture.

Summary

While the APT approach to managing pain represents a shift away from simple categories or dichotomies of patients, this chapter has outlined some categorizations that are relatively easy to consider but may have important influence over how you proceed. None of these by themselves are diagnostic, prognostic or theranostic categories. Rather we've framed them as considerations that should affect how you interpret the results of your assessments, if not affect how you choose them. An important note here that is worthy of specific consideration is this: the radar plot and patient phenotyping are only relevant *after* serious comorbidities have been adequately cleared and the patient has been deemed suitable for non-urgent medical or rehabilitation care. There are existing decision tools, such as the Canadian C-Spine Rule, the American College of Radiology Appropriateness Criteria, and a host of others (e.g. the Nexus criteria, Ottawa Ankle Rules) that should be cleared first (often by emergency medical personnel) before getting into any more detailed assessment and treatment. The radar plot comes into the picture usually at the first visit to a rehabilitation professional such as a physical therapist or possibly by a general medicine practitioner, and only after red flags have been ruled out as best they can. The flow diagram in Figure 5.2 provides a graphical description of where this kind of assessment fits in terms of the standard flow of a patient through the healthcare system.

After we explore prognosis further in Chapter 5, the subsequent sections of the book begin with the idea of a 'go-to toolbox', with each chapter then describing one of the seven domains of the radar plot. A recurrent theme is that we are endorsing a general framework rather than a hard and fast clinical practice rule. In all cases, you as the clinician should have confidence in harnessing your knowledge of the best available evidence, your experiences and intuitions with the patient in front of you, and that individual patient's values, beliefs and expectations when choosing the most appropriate way forward.

References

Bartley, E. J., Fillingim, R. B., 2013. Sex differences in pain: a brief review of clinical and experimental findings. *British Journal of Anaesthesia* 111 (1):52–8.

Chen, E. H., Shofer, F. S., Dean, A. J., et al., 2008. Gender disparity in analgesic treatment of emergency department patients with acute abdominal pain. *Academic Emergency Medicine: Official Journal of the Society for Academic Emergency Medicine* 15 (5):414–8.

Elliott, J. M., Dewald, J. P., Hornby, T. G., et al., 2014. Mechanisms underlying chronic whiplash: contributions from an incomplete spinal cord injury? *Pain Medicine* 15 (11):1938–44.

Foa, E. B., Cashman, L., Jaycox, L., et al., 1997. The validation of a self-report measures of posttraumatic stress disorder: the Posttraumatic Diagnostic Scale. *Psychological Assessment* 9:445–51.

Hill, J. C., Dunn, K. M., Main, C. J., et al., 2010. Subgrouping low back pain: a comparison of the STarT Back Tool with the Orebro Musculoskeletal Pain Screening Questionnaire. *European Journal of Pain* 14 (1):83–9.

Hoffmann, D. E., Tarzian, A. J., 2001. The girl who cried pain: a bias against women in the treatment of pain. *The Journal of Law, Medicine & Ethics: A Journal of the American Society of Law, Medicine & Ethics* 29 (1):13–27.

Horowitz, M., Wilner, N., Alvarez, W., 1979. Impact of Event Scale: A measure of subjective stress. *Psychosomatic Medicine* 41:209–18.

Kelly, J., Ritchie, C., Sterling, M., 2017. Clinical prediction rules for prognosis and treatment prescription in neck pain: A systematic review. *Musculoskeletal Science and Practice* 27:155–64.

Schuh-Hofer, S., Wodarski, R., Pfau, D. B., et al., 2013. One night of total sleep deprivation promotes a state of generalized hyperalgesia: A surrogate pain model to study the relationship of insomnia and pain. *Pain* 154 (9):1613–21.

Scott, D., Jull, G., Sterling, M., 2005. Widespread sensory hypersensitivity is a feature of chronic whiplash-associated disorder but not chronic idiopathic neck pain. *The Clinical Journal of Pain* 21 (2):175–81.

Walton, D. M., Macdermid, J. C., Nielson, W., et al., 2011. A descriptive study of pressure pain threshold at 2 standardized sites in people with acute or subacute neck pain. *The Journal of Orthopaedic and Sports Physical Therapy* 41 (9):651–7.

Walton, D. M., Balsor, B., Etruw, E., 2012. Exploring the causes of neck pain and disability as perceived by those who experience the condition: a mixed-methods study. *ISRN Rehabilitation* 2012:1–7.

Walton, D. M., Macdermid, J. C., Giorgianni, A. A., et al., 2013. Risk factors for persistent problems following acute whiplash injury: Update of a systematic review and meta-analysis. *Journal of Orthopaedic and Sports Physical Therapy* 43 (2):31–43.

Weathers, F.W., Litz, B.T., Herman, D.S., et al., 1993. The PTSD Checklist (PCL): reliability, validity, and diagnostic utility. Paper presented at the Annual Meeting of International Society for Traumatic Stress Studies, San Antonio, TX, October, 1993, 2, 90–92.

5

Understanding Prognosis, or 'How to Predict the Future'

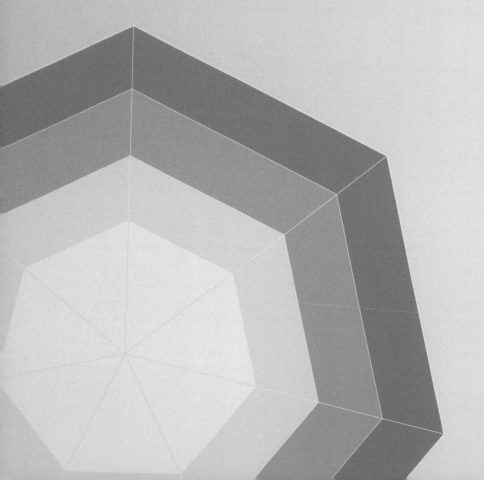

The 'P' in the 'APT' acronym stands for 'Predict' and is a core component to the APT framework. It can also standard for 'prognosis', and we find the concept of a prognosis-based approach to assessment and evaluation quite attractive. Traditional clinical approaches have focused on evaluation procedures to 'find' the culprit (sometimes referred to as the 'tissue at fault') and then presenting interventions strategies aimed at 'fixing' the tissue. This model has become problematic for many reasons, one reason being the notion that there is some version of 'normal' that all tissues should approximate, and under this model it is the clinician's job to normalize those tissues. We can see the often-harmful implications of this way of thinking across several disciplines. The first has been the generation of a culture that appears to hold these assumptions of 'normality' as truths, and that anything that deviates from normal must therefore be problematic and cured. Those in the pain education field have been working for the past 20 years to undo the harm that has been created, for some people, through the endorsement of this way of thinking. The whole mentality of 'I hurt, therefore my tissues must be damaged' (hurt = harm) is likely an offshoot of the traditional 'tissue-at-fault' models of clinical practice. On the other end of that issue is the growing body of research findings indicating 'abnormal' tissue or joint loads, mechanics or integrity (e.g. diagnostic imaging or movement analyses) are rarely and unreliably related to the patient's complaints. That is, the evidence of what would normally be considered tissue damage without related pain, or pain without related tissue damage. While newer evidence is starting to show that when imaging findings are interpreted in different ways (Elliott et al., 2018) an association with clinical symptoms (pain and function) may well exist, these are still some way off from being routine practice.

One way we have reconciled the seeming discordance between tissue 'normality' and clinical signs and symptoms in the APT framework is through the radar plot concept, that recognizes the experience of pain can be driven by several different domains. This is an important departure from traditional focus on just one domain (nociceptive/physiological) that relates to tissue integrity or mechanics. This approach to multi-domain phenotyping allows multiple drivers in the same person that all interact to collectively explain a patient's pain experience. In this way, a primary nociceptive driver can co-exist in the presence of central nociplastic change that facilitates or even amplifies the 'harm' message as it ascends through the central nervous system (a process some might call 'central sensitization'). If one were to focus only on finding the problematic tissue, then clinical tests may well be difficult to interpret in the presence of several other pain drivers.

Another novel component of this framework is this emphasis on predicting outcomes, which can be summed up this way: if the likely outcome (prognosis) of a patient's condition is good, then let nature take its course and keep your intervention/interference to a minimum, whereas if the likely outcome is poor, then do your best to determine *why* and intervene in a judicious, targeted fashion. Where possible, the intention is to mitigate the risks and improve the likelihood of a good outcome. Simple right?

Predicting outcomes

The concept of predicting outcomes is going to take different forms under different contexts, most notably the acute vs. chronic dichotomy from Chapter 4. To understand why, it is first important to understand the nature of such predictions. Most readers will be familiar with the term *prognosis*, which has become a term used to encapsulate all such outcome predictions, though not always correctly. In its simplest form, the term 'prognosis' is a prediction based on the most likely outcome of expected events. It can be used in business, economics, law, or many other fields, but in our case, we'll focus on prognosis as it relates to health and illness, and all the in-between happenings of those extremes. In common lexicon, when someone asks 'What's *my* prognosis?' they're quite likely asking: what can I expect regarding the short-, intermediate- or long-term course of *my* disease? How likely is it that this will get worse or better? Do *I* need treatment and how likely is it that the treatments available, and delivered, will improve *my* outcome? While these all seem related, when we break it down, we see that these are all different questions that require different concepts of predicting the future.

What can I expect regarding the short, intermediate, or long-term course of my disease? How likely is it that this will get worse or better? To answer these questions, a clinician needs a considerable amount of information. They need to know:

- What is currently known about the *natural course* of this condition or disease? That is, without any treatment provided, what can the *average*[1] patient expect in the short, medium, and long term?

- How was that information derived, and on what type of patient sample or population?

- What outcome was used in the research to derive the natural course, and is that outcome relevant for my patient?

- Does my patient have similar characteristics to those samples, such that I can generalize research findings to the patient in front of me?

- Does my patient have any protective or risk factors that mean I should adjust the known natural course (trajectory) up or down? If so, by how much?

- What is currently known about the *clinical course* of this condition or disease? That is, when managed according to current best practices, what can the *average* patient expect in the short, medium, and long term?

[1] Remember that an average is only an average because scores fall on both sides of that number. In many studies, no single patient falls right on the average.

As you can see, 'What's my prognosis?' is not a terribly easy question to answer. Even those of us who spend our days researching in the field of prognosis and longitudinal modeling have difficulty with many of these questions. When we talk about predicting outcomes, what outcome are we trying to predict? Death? Discharge? Remission? Return to work? Complete recovery? If complete recovery, what does that mean, and does it mean the same thing to all people? What kinds of people do we want to follow in our studies? Should we embrace the messiness of humans (including all their confounders) and follow all people with a condition, or should we try to homogenize the sample by only following those with the condition of interest but otherwise good health? Do those people even exist? If so, how and when do they end up in a clinical practice, and would knowing more about them be of any clinical use? If we just accept all comers, how can we tell if the outcome is just due to the natural course of the condition of interest or any number of other health-related comorbidities? Can we ask our participants to avoid interventions or activities that might affect the natural course? Is it ethical to do so? If not, can we provide the same treatment to everyone to reduce confounders? Is that a fair representation of the clinical course? Does the type of intervention that we deliver even matter? AHHHHH!!!

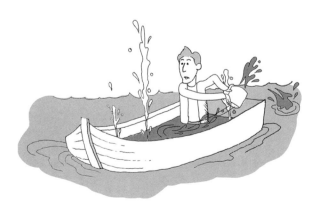

Clearly, the field of predicting outcomes is messy, difficult to understand, and filled with divergent findings. However, while difficult, we can't simply ignore the issue(s) as these are critically important for making treatment decisions. Going back to an earlier point, the APT framework proposes that, following a sound assessment including a focus on those person-level factors that are likely to affect recovery and prognosis, if the patient is likely to recover well without (or perhaps despite) intervention, then this is good news and should be relayed to the patient as such. Clinicians in this case, we suggest, should take a hands-off approach and let the natural course of recovery occur. If the risk-based assessment reveals a greater likelihood of a more problematic course, then the clinician should also know this and, if possible, be prepared to intervene based on the known risk factors present. So, we cannot throw our hands in the air and proclaim that predicting outcomes is too difficult. After all, it's precisely this type of information that patients are most commonly seeking.

Prognosis vs. theranosis

For the purposes of making this exercise more palatable, we're going to break the notion of predicting outcomes into two different concepts; one that is more relevant in the *acute* stage of injury or pain, and the other that is more relevant to the *chronic* stage (though both will hold relevance in both stages). The two concepts are *prognosis* and *theranosis*. We're going to define these in this way:

> **Prognosis**: The expected *trend* in the course of a condition as indicated by outcome 'X' ('X' in this case being whatever outcome is meaningful to you and your patient). This can be short, medium, or long term, which for our purposes we're going to broadly define as 6 weeks (short term), 3 months (medium term), and 12 months (long term); these are somewhat arbitrary but also in keeping with much of the prognostic research for many musculoskeletal pain conditions. So, by classifying things this way we can lean on what evidence exists. Key to prognosis then, is having a good handle on not only the condition being asked about, but on the outcome being predicted and the time frame over which the prediction makes the most sense.

> **Theranosis**: A portmanteau of 'therapy' and 'diagnosis/prognosis', theranosis is the predicted response to a single administration, or a course, of a specific treatment. If prognosis is an overall umbrella term for 'predicting an outcome', theranosis is a sub-domain of prognosis,

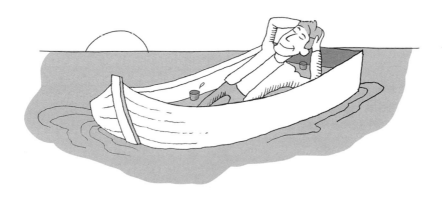

focusing more on the 'clinical course', or the anticipated outcomes if treatment X is provided to patient Y. If the treatment (therapy) is most commonly delivered as a course or package of treatment, then theranosis and prognosis start to overlap somewhat. But in the case of theranosis we can also ask: what is the most likely effect on this patient's health status after a single administration of this treatment? In this way theranosis does not rely as much on the long-term data collection procedures as prognosis does, and the study design is more likely to be a clinical trial rather than a purely observational cohort study. That said, most journals will not publish studies that do NOT include some degree of at least medium-term follow-up, so that information may still be available.

In practical terms, prognosis is more relevant to those in the acute stage of pain or injury, simply because acute conditions tend to be very labile in their presentations early on while chronic pain conditions are generally more stable. To put it another way, while prognosis is still valuable for people with chronic pain, the target of the prognosis needs to shift since, clearly, the prognosis for persistent pain has already proven itself to not be good. Theranosis therefore holds arguably *more* relevance for those with chronic pain conditions: 'If I were to engage in your offered treatment, what is the anticipated effect on my pain or disability?' Again, this is not to say that theranosis does *not* hold relevance in the acute context: especially for those who are deemed to be at higher risk for non-recovery, it would be good to know how the anticipated trajectory (clinical course) may *shift* if a particular treatment is administered early.

Practical applications

Let's see how these concepts play out in practice. Having focused so far on neck and low back pain,

we'll continue to use these conditions to frame this discussion. Fortunately, these conditions are also where we can find the most evidence on prognosis. In 2010, researchers from Australia followed 155 people with acute (<4 weeks) traumatic neck pain (whiplash) for up to one year capturing outcomes at baseline, and again three, six and twelve months later (Sterling et al., 2010). In this case, the outcomes were functional impairment as measured using the common Neck Disability Index (NDI) and post-traumatic distress symptoms measured using the Post-Traumatic Distress Diagnostic Scale (PDS). Using a statistical technique known as *latent growth curve analysis* (used to identify similar 'clusters' of trajectories within a large group of data), these authors identified three trajectories for both of the outcomes followed: a mildly affected/rapid recovery group that represented 40–45% of the sample, a moderately affected/moderate recovery group that represented another 39–43% of the sample, and a severely affected/non-recovery group of 16–17% (Fig. 5.1). In 2016 another group of Australian researchers followed a large group of 1585 patients with acute (<6 weeks) low back pain, capturing outcomes weekly for 12 weeks (Downie et al., 2016). In this case the outcome being followed was pain intensity on a common 0-10 Numeric Rating Scale. Despite the different conditions (neck vs. low back pain) and different outcomes, these authors found largely similar results: a group who started off with mild pain and recovered well representing 36% of the sample, a couple of groups who started off more affected and recovered more slowly or incompletely representing about 48% of the sample (combined), and then a couple of groups who started off with intense pain and reported either ongoing severe pain or fluctuating pain representing a combined 16% of the sample. Using data from our own longitudinal acute pain cohort studies, we conducted a similar analysis on a mixed sample of 235 people presenting to a non-emergency urgent care center

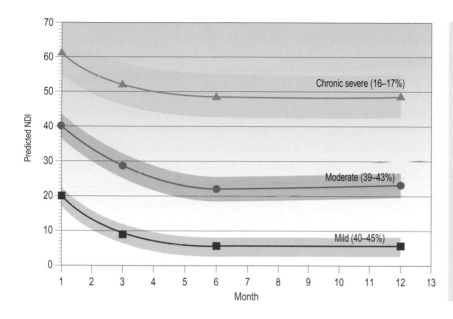

Figure 5.1
Predicted NDI trajectories with color-coded 95% confidence limits and predicted probability of group membership (%). (Reproduced with permission from Sterling, M., Hendrikz, J., Kenardy, J., 2010. Compensation claim lodgement and health outcome developmental trajectories following whiplash injury: A prospective study. *Pain* 150 (1):22–8.)

with non-catastrophic neck, low back, upper or lower extremity injuries within two weeks of injury. We captured several outcomes; the primary being pain-related interference measured with the common Brief Pain Inventory (BPI). We also found three trajectories that best described the data though the shapes in our mixed musculoskeletal trauma sample were slightly different: a mild baseline and smooth recovery group (76%), a high baseline but rapid recovery group we're calling the 'resilient' group (11%), and a high baseline with no or little recovery group we'll call the 'chronic' group (11%). Of note, when we separated the entire database into those with axial (neck or low back) injuries and those with peripheral (upper or lower extremity) injuries, the proportions in our axial group were similar to that which Sterling and Downie previously found, with 15% in the chronic group. So, taken together, and in light of several other such studies with similar results, it seems we can generally assume most people will take one of at least three trajectories following non-catastrophic musculoskeletal trauma: fairly mild acute symptoms with a generally good

outcome (~45% of people), an initially more moderate and slower, possibly incomplete, recovery course (~40% of people), and then a group who starts out more severely affected and never really recovers (~15% of people). In none of the studies described were the participants restricted from receiving care, but in a somewhat damning commentary on many approaches to acute pain management and rehabilitation, it seems the nature or type of intervention doesn't really matter. In the study by Downie and colleagues on those 1585 people with low back pain, paracetamol as an intervention was no better than placebo.

The next question is regarding the factors that are known to influence those three (or perhaps more) recovery trajectories. As astute readers may have picked up by now, one of the most consistent predictors of the course of a condition is how severe it is at the outset. High pain intensity is, and has long-been, a strong predictor of poor pain recovery; high self-rated disability predicts poor disability recovery; high post-traumatic distress symptoms predict poor emotional recovery; and so on. One thing we can say with reasonable confidence is that the best predictor of any outcome in the future is the intensity of that same predictor at baseline. There are both conceptual and statistical reasons for that, but when you step back and think about it for a minute, it just makes common sense. If I were to predict whether you'd be working a year from now, the first question I'd ask is whether you have a job now. It's great when common sense helps out. But there do appear to be some other factors that may predict the trajectory beyond their entry point into the clinic.

Back in 2009 we published a review and statistical pooling technique (a 'meta-analysis') of prognosis and risk factors in whiplash (Walton et al., 2009), and then updated that in 2013 (Walton et al., 2013). Some other groups have since performed similar analyses, and the results have been fairly consistent. As expected, higher ratings on initial pain or disability indexes are consistent predictors of high ratings six or twelve months later. We were also able to find cut scores on some of those tools that earned people membership to the high-risk categories, and those have also been fairly consistent. For a simple 0-10 pain intensity rating scale, a score of 6/10 or higher in the acute stage of injury appears to be problematic, while a score >30% on a neck-related disability scale like the NDI should also 'raise an eyebrow'. Interestingly, this is about the same threshold score that Ritchie and colleagues found when deriving and validating their clinical prediction rule for estimating recovery trajectories in an independent sample of people with whiplash (Ritchie et al., 2013; Fig. 5.2).

The results are fairly similar in low back pain, where more severe pain and disability early on are predictive of the slower or incomplete recovery trajectories. But what about other domains such as those shown on the radar plot? It seems those also have some, if not a lot, of predictive value. In the structural/nociceptive

domain, there is increasing evidence that poor muscle quality (as quantified using fatty infiltration) is a risk factor for poorer recovery in neck (Elliott et al., 2011; Elliott et al., 2015) low back (Hancock et al., 2017), and rotator cuff injuries (Raman et al., 2017). In the psychological domains (cognitive or emotional), we and others have consistently found that higher scores on scales that measure things like catastrophizing (an exaggerated negative orientation towards pain), depression, or post-traumatic distress all seem to be more common in the high risk/non-recovery groups. Dedicated tools for prognosis are also now available, such as Hill's Keele STarT Back tool (Hill et al., 2004), and our very own Traumatic Injuries Distress Scale (Walton et al., 2016), both of which tap primarily cognitive domains. In the central and sensorimotor domains, widespread mechanical hyperalgesia (most commonly measured using a pressure-measuring device with a small rubber tip called an 'algometer'), and hypersensitivity to cold also seem to be signs of potential problems (Walton et al., 2011; Sterling, 2010; Elliott et al., 2009). In the socioenvironmental domain, there has been some evidence, though it is somewhat conflicting, if not controversial (see Chapter 4), that women, people from lower educational or socioeconomic backgrounds, and middle-aged people (35–55 years old) are more likely to be in the poor recovery group. Social determinants of health have become so important that an entire academic discipline is now dedicated to their study. There's even a 'broken window' theory, which suggests that living in a neighborhood with visible signs of crime, anti-social behavior, and civil disorder create more crime and disorder (and likely influence health and well-being). A fascinating connection between ZIP-codes and human health has interested researchers for many years. So much so, that Dr. Francis Collins, Director of the National Institutes of Health, recently noted that ZIP code at birth should be referred to as our ZNA; the blueprint for our behavioral and psychosocial makeup (Schwartz & Hirsch, 2015).

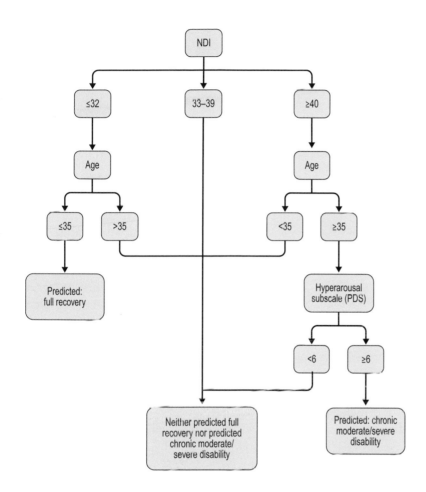

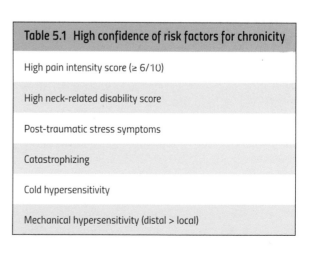

Figure 5.2
A derived clinical prediction rule to predict both full recovery and persistent moderate/severe disability after an acute whiplash injury. (Reproduced with permission from Ritchie, C., Hendrikz, J., Kenardy, J., Sterling, M., 2013. Derivation of a clinical prediction rule to identify both chronic moderate/severe disability and full recovery following whiplash injury. *Pain* 154 (10):2198–206.)

Being involved in litigation related to the injury seems to be a factor that veers those who were otherwise on a good trajectory towards the slower recovery curves, while those who were already in the severe/non-recovery groups aren't affected by opening an injury claim (Sterling et al., 2010). Table 5.1 shows some of the more consistent risk factors for poor prognosis especially in neck pain. Importantly, the radar plot domains have been chosen not only for their potential ability to guide treatment decisions, but as you've hopefully just noted, also because they hold value for creating a *prognostic phenotype*.

Table 5.1 High confidence of risk factors for chronicity
High pain intensity score (≥ 6/10)
High neck-related disability score
Post-traumatic stress symptoms
Catastrophizing
Cold hypersensitivity
Mechanical hypersensitivity (distal > local)

This brings us to theranosis. As mentioned, we believe theranosis is *more* relevant for chronic conditions than acute conditions – mainly because we have so little evidence to rely on for management of acute musculoskeletal conditions. This is part of the reason why the APT philosophy focuses so much on deep phenotyping and clinical reasoning – *conduct a sound assessment, predict the likelihood of recovery, and intervene accordingly.* As we discussed in Chapter 2, few clinical research studies are designed to allow consideration of so many different factors at once in their analyses, meaning you as the clinician must rely on your skills, observations and interpretations, knowledge, creativity and clinical reasoning. This is certainly not to suggest that all is lost. While you may not be able to lean heavily on evidence, clinical reasoning and common sense can indeed help, and the radar plot can offer some justification for your treatment decisions. Does the patient appear to be harboring strong negative misconceptions about the nature of his/her pain that you believe may be contributing to that very pain and disability? Then, it stands to reason that a good educational intervention would be indicated to break what appears to be a vicious cycle. Does there appear to be a strong driver of excessive

mechanical load on a sensitive tissue? Then perhaps a splinting or other unloading intervention makes sense. We will be providing this type of guidance for treatment decisions throughout the domain-specific chapters in the second part of this book.

Summary

We have presented and delved somewhat deeply into the concepts of prognosis and theranosis. We have further implied that prognosis or risk-based assessment is more relevant for those in the acute stage of injury or pain, while theranostic assessment is more relevant in the chronic stage, though both hold relevance regardless of symptom duration and interventions. Finally, we have described how the radar plot can be used for both prognostic and theranostic decisions by creating an appropriate profile of the patient and their pain experience.

Moving into the next sections of this book we begin laying out concrete examples of the different domains of the radar plot and how those can be assessed and, where possible, quantified in the clinical environment.

References

Downie, A. S., Hancock, M. J., Rzewuska, M., et al., 2016. Trajectories of acute low back pain: a latent class growth analysis. *Pain* 157 (1):225–34.

Elliott, J., Sterling, M., Noteboom, J.T., et al., 2009. The clinical presentation of chronic whiplash and the relationship to findings of MRI fatty infiltrates in the cervical extensor musculature: a preliminary investigation. *European Spine Journal* 18(9):1371–8.

Elliott, J., Pedler, A., Kenardy, J., et al., 2011. The temporal development of fatty infiltrates in the neck muscles following whiplash injury: an association with pain and posttraumatic stress. *PloS One* 6 (6):e21194.

Elliott, J. M., Courtney, D. M., Rademaker, A., et al., 2015. The rapid and progressive degeneration of the cervical multifidus in whiplash. *Spine* 40 (12): E694–E700.

Elliott, J. M., Hancock, M. J., Crawford, R. J., et al., 2018. Advancing imaging technologies for patients with spinal pain: with a focus on whiplash injury. *Spine Journal* 18 (8):1489–97.

Hancock, M. J., Kjaer, P., Kent, P., et al., 2017. Is the number of different MRI findings more strongly associated with low back pain than single MRI findings? *Spine* 42 (17):1283–8.

Hill, J., Lewis, M., Papageorgiou, A. C., et al., 2004. Predicting persistent neck pain: a 1-year follow-up of a population cohort. *Spine* 29 (15):1648–54.

Raman, J., Walton, D., MacDermid, J. C., et al., 2017. Predictors of outcomes after rotator cuff repair—a meta-analysis. *Journal of Hand Therapy* 30 (3):276–92.

Ritchie, C., Hendrikz, J., Kenardy, J., et al., 2013. Derivation of a clinical prediction rule to identify both chronic moderate/severe disability and full recovery following whiplash injury. *Pain* 154 (10):2198–2206.

Schwartz, B. S., Hirsch, A., 2015. The key to your health could be in your ZIP code. Available at: https://theconversation.com/the-key-to-your-health-could-be-in-your-zip-code-46304.

Sterling, M., 2010. Differential development of sensory hypersensitivity and a measure of spinal cord hyperexcitability following whiplash injury. *Pain* 150 (3):501–6.

Sterling, M., Hendrikz, J., Kenardy, J., 2010. Compensation claim lodgement and health outcome developmental trajectories following whiplash injury: a prospective study. *Pain* 150 (1):22–8.

Walton, D. M., Pretty, J., MacDermid, J. C., et al., 2009. Risk factors for persistent problems following whiplash injury: results of a systematic review and meta-analysis. *Journal of Orthopaedic and Sports Physical Therapy* 39 (5):334–50.

Walton, D. M., Macdermid, J. C., Nielson, W., et al., 2011. Pressure pain threshold testing demonstrates predictive ability in people with acute whiplash. *The Journal of Orthopaedic and Sports Physical Therapy* 41 (9):658–65.

Walton, D. M., Macdermid, J. C., Giorgianni, A. A., et al., 2013. Risk factors for persistent problems following acute whiplash injury: update of a systematic review and meta-analysis. *The Journal of Orthopaedic and Sports Physical Therapy* 43 (2):31–43.

Walton, D. M., Krebs, D., Moulden, D., et al., 2016. The Traumatic Injuries Distress Scale: a new tool that quantifies distress and has predictive validity with patient-reported outcomes. *Journal of Orthopedic and Sports Physical Therapy* 46 (10):920–8.

6

Creating Your 'Go-To' Toolbox

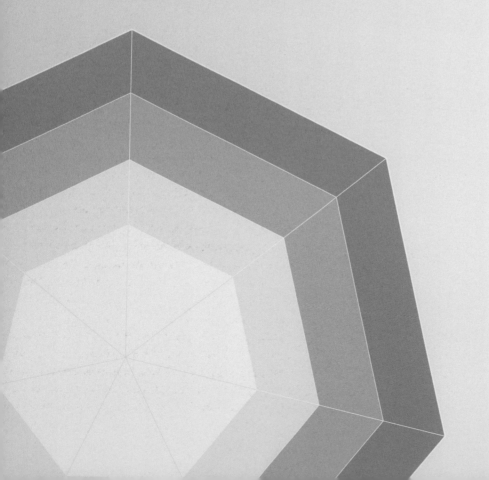

One of the ways to limit the total number of scales or tests is to begin with a simple three- or four-domain set of tools that you can have all patients complete either while in the waiting room of your clinic or even at home before they arrive for their first appointment. If this 'go-to toolbox' is chosen carefully and with intention, it should be both generic enough to be applicable across conditions (regardless of your patient's primary complaint) yet provide rich information across several of the radar plot domains to direct further assessments. In this way, you can orient your initial assessments towards domains that appear to be especially problematic for your patient while potentially ruling out other domains that do not appear to be strong drivers of the patient's pain experience and can therefore be given lower priority.

We recognize it is not easy to identify patient self-report tools that fit nicely within this go-to toolbox, but fortunately we've been in this field a long time and have identified a number that fit for us, and hopefully for you too. Our primary goal in providing this information is not to endorse or set a hard and fast rule about the tools you *must* or even *ought to* use, but to provide insights into how we go about choosing our go-to tools. We recognize that new tools are becoming available all the time, and that as we enter an era of machine learning and artificially intelligent (AI) predictive algorithms, the day of the simple pencil-and-paper form is very likely drawing to a close. But, current trends tell us that clinicians and patients will continue to favor such 'analog' tools for another decade or so (into the mid-2020s) so we are reinforcing those examples here. We do hope however that readers will not shy away from AI-enhanced decision-making tools as they come available, and we believe the insights we are providing here will still be relevant for selecting appropriate tools and questions even as we progress further into the digital revolution and the age of knowledge.

Considerations for choosing a tool for your 'go-to' toolbox

When considering what to include in your go-to toolbox, which itself is intended more as a quick screen to help focus your assessment rather than a detailed set of diagnostic tools, there are several considerations. Tools that you want to consider for your personal toolbox should:

1. **Be brief.** No one wants to spend a half hour reading instructions on how to circle numbers on a page, and the longer people go at it, the less time they spend considering each answer and hence the less valid their responses start to become. The entire toolbox should be able to be completed in no more than 5 minutes by someone with at least high-school fluency in the language and no other learning or cognitive deficits. Depending on the nature of the questions some may require more time to reflect upon and answer than others (e.g. opinion-based scales generally take longer to answer than do frequency-based scales), but as a general rule of thumb you can estimate about 10 seconds per question on a questionnaire. So, a 10-item questionnaire should be easily completable within about 1 minute 40 seconds. If we use our 5-minute total time guide, then that's about 30 total questions across all the scales in your toolbox that should be the upper limit of acceptable to most patients.

2. **Be generic.** As a busy clinician you don't want to have different tool sets for people with neck pain, low back pain, knee pain, shoulder pain,

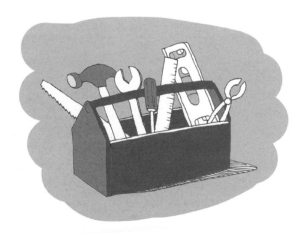

acute pain, chronic pain, traumatic pain, non-traumatic pain, and so on. And the more such tool sets you have, the more likely you or someone else (e.g. front desk staff) will choose the wrong one. A 'set it and forget it' approach is far more useful here from a quick screening perspective. This means that the tools you choose for your go-to toolbox need to be relevant across a wide range of clinical conditions, patients, and settings. This is not always easy, and some tools that are meant to be generic are not always as generic as they first seem. For example the Brief Pain Inventory (BPI) (Cleeland & Ryan, 1994), which will feature later on, is widely endorsed as a generic patient-reported outcome for capturing pain severity and pain-related interference regardless of the region of injury, or even the nature of the condition (it was originally developed for use in cancer pain though has since been applied to several pain-related conditions). However, previous authors have found it doesn't work equally well across all patient populations.

One of the interference questions pertains to walking ability, which would not apply to someone who uses a wheelchair for mobility. Barney and colleagues (2018) tackled this problem by revising the item to read "mobility (ability to get around)". Similarly, if the presenting and primary complaint is a shoulder or neck problem, then asking about interference with walking may not be relevant. In this case not only is it forcing the patient to answer a question that may have no bearing on their condition, but it also means that the responsiveness of the scale overall is decreased, as this question is unlikely to ever change no matter how effective the shoulder treatment you administer. Another item on the BPI pertains to interference with work, that may not be immediately relevant to all respondents, especially those who don't work in the traditional sense or are retired. Darnall and Sazie (2012) ran into this problem when studying the impact of pain in incarcerated women. They solved the problem by removing items referring to 'work' and 'sex' to fit the study population.

While the BPI is one of the most widely recognized generic pain tools in the world, the point of these examples is that even tools that are widely used and meant to be generic still present challenges for certain groups of patients. Regardless of the tool(s) you choose, it is difficult to get around another issue that most share, and that is the general assumption that all items on a scale are equally important to all people. We will explore this concept of individual item importance later in this chapter, but for now we believe the concept of weighting functional scale items by importance is something that is well worth exploring further, for both clinicians and researchers.

3. **Provide rich information.** While the Brief Pain Inventory may present some challenges for some patient groups, it is also useful in that the short form of the tool is brief (11 total items to score) and provides standardized metrics for pain severity, physical interference, affective interference, and sleep interference (Walton et al., 2016). In fact, the BPI also includes a body diagram for pain location, a space to describe the medications the patient is taking for their pain, and an indication of how effective those have been. So, this is an example of a single tool that provides a lot of information, and even with just these domains available you can start to build the beginnings of a radar plot for your patient. The BPI is certainly not the only tool to have this quality, and as you'll see below, we prefer a more detailed body diagram to the one

the BPI has to offer. The important contribution of these scales is that if used properly they can provide foundation for triangulating the patient's pain experience across the radar plot domains before you even lay eyes on the patient themselves.

4. **Have at least some evidence to support its validity.** Validation of a measurement tool is a strange and nebulous idea, the finer nuances of which are beyond the purpose of this book. Suffice it to say for now that validation is a process rather than an end-point, and that no self-report tool (and most physical assessment tests) should ever be described as 'validated'. Rather, you want to find tools that at least have *adequate evidence* (in your mind) that they are providing accurate representations of the underlying construct (the 'real' reality in critical realist terms) that they're meant to be measuring. That said, even adequate evidence is an intentionally soft goal that leaves plenty of room for your own interpretation. At the height of the evidence-based practice movement in the late 1990s/early 2000s, clinicians were told to *only* use tools that had been validated on the specific patient population to which their patient belonged. While this is a sound theoretical approach, it led to widespread clinical decision-making paralysis as there were (and are) very few tools in existence that could meet such stringent criteria.

Thankfully, in most circles evidence-*based* practice has been replaced with the concept of evidence-*informed* practice (EIP). EIP still places high priority on sound empirical research and the use of best available knowledge, but also gives equal weight to clinician experience and patient values. This means that 'adequately valid' scales are at least findable, and we can accept that validity comes in many different flavors towards facilitating practice decisions rather than complicating them.

In some cases, you as the clinician may be satisfied as long as the scale has *face validity* (that is, the questions being asked of the patient appear to be tapping the underlying construct of interest). Face validity is widely considered one of the weakest forms of scale validation but is still an important step. For quick screening such as the tools in your go-to toolbox, you may decide that face validity is enough for you to adopt a scale because the items are otherwise important but not likely to influence your clinical decisions. On the other end of the 'validity' continuum is *criterion-related* validity; the degree to which the results of a tool can be taken to reflect (i.e. can substitute for) a more burdensome 'gold standard'. If the gold standard is considered to provide the 'real reality' (or at least accurately captures the empirical reality) of the construct being measured, then any new tool that is intended to tap that same construct should be compared against that standard. This is a difficult target for intensely personal experiences like pain (or love, guilt, sadness, etc.) because no gold standard for comparison exists. As a result, few pain-related tools ever really satisfy the requirements for criterion-related validity. Other types of validity including concurrent (convergent/divergent), predictive, discriminative, or known-groups, are also important dependent on the intended use of the tool.

We are intentionally not being prescriptive in stating just *how* valid a scale needs to be as that would be a slippery slope we wish not to travel. Rather, we endorse common clinical sense in choosing appropriate tools (that is, read the tool and ensure the items at least *make sense*). This common sense approach is one we've endorsed previously (Walton, 2015). What we'd strongly caution against however is to simply make up your own questions and have patients complete them without at least doing some preliminary psychometric work – measurement is a powerful thing, and so poor tools could lead to poor treatment. At the same time, we don't believe you should avoid a scale altogether simply because it hasn't been rigorously tested and scrutinized in your specific patient population. Common sense should prevail here.

So, the suggested criteria for your go-to toolbox tools are that they: 1) are brief; 2) are generic; 3) provide rich information; and 4) have at least some evidence to support their appropriate measurement properties. There are several tools that could fit these criteria, but, based on our years of clinical practice and measurement research, we provide a set of tools for you to consider. You may wish to start with these then adapt them as new information comes along or create an entirely new toolbox that is unique to your setting. As long as you can follow the general spirit of the go-to toolbox, then the choice of the actual tool(s) is up to you.

One final caveat here is that all of the tools listed in Table 6.1 are freely available for use by individual clinicians without requiring permission from a copyright holder. Please be sure to observe copyright laws when you are selecting tools as we know of some clinicians who have gotten themselves in trouble by using (and posting on their clinics' websites) tools that were in fact copyright protected and were not freely available.

The three tools (Body Diagram, BIPQ, BPI) comprise 22 total items and can be easily completed in 5 minutes, but together provide a wealth of information as a first-pass screen and the beginnings of your triangulation and phenotyping exercise.

As detailed in the 'alternatives' section of Table 6.1, many other tools exist that could also fill these roles. Some readers will be familiar with the Patient-Specific Functional Scale for example (PSFS). This has been described as either a 3- or 5-item patient-centered scale in which the patients themselves create the items informed by their specific functional goals. So, a patient with ankle pain may describe functional goals of walking, getting up from the floor, and skiing. The clinician records those and then asks the patient to rate their current satisfaction with their function on each of those items on a standard 0–10 numeric rating scale, where presumably the goal would be to hit a '10 = fully functional' on each one. This is a nice idea for a clinical tool though has been something of a nightmare to empirically study as everyone's scale is different, so group averages are awfully hard to interpret. The Canadian Occupational Performance Measure (COPM) (Law et al., 1990) is a similar concept, though this one includes two separate scales for each patient-generated item, an importance scale and a satisfaction scale. As mentioned, the addition of importance is an interesting idea, and has remained under-researched owing to the challenges of different patient-generated scales. In 2015, we published a tool called the Satisfaction and Recovery Index (SRI) (Walton et al., 2014) that is conceptualized as patient-centric but more standardized than the PSFS or COPM. To create this scale we used information from patients with chronic pain, asking them how the recovered version of themselves would be different from the current version (Walton et al., 2013). From that, we created nine generic health-related satisfaction items (plus one attention check item) that ask patients to provide two ratings for each: an importance score, and a satisfaction score. Scoring is a little more complex on this one but not terribly difficult, and a free spreadsheet can be accessed from www.pirlresearch.com. The SRI provides

Table 6.1   A sample APT go-to toolbox

Tool	Brief description	What it can tell you
A detailed body diagram	Should provide either an androgynous line drawing of a body, or options for male and female line drawings, with views of the front, back, left and right sides, and detailed views of the hands, feet, and possibly face, head and genitals. Some are broken into regions to allow quantification, others are blank and wide open. We like ones that allow the patient to not only mark the area(s) of their body with pain, but also areas with other related symptoms like burning, radiation, numbness or prickling pains. A line drawing version is available on www.pirlresearch.com, or online interactive versions are available such as the PainQUILT maintained by McMaster University (Canada) at painquilt.com.	Several pieces of information are possible depending on the diagram you use. Primary and secondary areas of pain will help you focus your assessment, but also provide clues about whether the pain drivers are more likely peripheral nociception (localized discreet areas of pain) or central nociplastic (widespread and poorly defined pain). If other pain descriptors are included (e.g. burning, prickling, numbness) you may glean clues about the likelihood of peripheral neuropathy. If the diagram is broken into distinct regions, it is possible it could be used to calculate percent of body in pain and therefore used as a tool to evaluate treatment effectiveness, though responsiveness on most such tools is not strong.
The Brief Illness Perceptions Questionnaire	Created by Broadbent and colleagues (2006) and built upon Leventhal's Common Sense Model of Health and Illness Representations, the BIPQ in its original form is a 10-item questionnaire, comprising nine 0–10 numeric rating scales and one open-ended question on which patients are asked to describe the most likely drivers of their health condition from their own perspectives. The 0–10 scales are meant to be interpreted separately and tap into the domains of the Illness Representations model, including things such as intensity, expected duration, sense of control, understanding, emotional impact, sense of fragility, and confidence in treatment. An adapted version has been created that separates the symptom intensity item into two: one for number of symptoms and one for intensity of those symptoms that can be accessed at www.pirlresearch.com.	Each question conceivably provides valuable information on its own, so 10 or 11 pieces of information on a single tool. What are the patient's expectations of how long the condition will last? How confident are they that treatment will help? How concerned are they? How well do they understand their condition? How much of an emotional impact has it taken? Every one of these could lead to important additional questioning, and also provide pieces of evidence for your radar plot, this time more in the cognitive and emotional domains. Generally speaking, any item rated 7 or higher (or 3 or lower for the 'good' items) is worthy of further consideration. We used the BIPQ to identify 3 subgroups of patients with neck pain: low, moderate and highly distressed, that would either add to or reduce the emotional domains of the radar plot (Walton et al., 2015b). We also found that those who endorsed trauma as a primary cause of their symptoms were more likely to be distressed (Walton et al., 2012) again adding additional information to your patient profiling exercise.

continued

Table 6.1 A sample APT go-to toolbox *continued*		
Tool	**Brief description**	**What it can tell you**
The Brief Pain Inventory	The BPI is a generic and well-known pain severity and interference scale that has ample evidence of adequate validity and has been translated into many languages. Being a widely-used scale there are plenty of existing data against which you can compare your patient if you so desire. The original includes a low-resolution body diagram, a section to enter medications used and their effectiveness, and two quantifiable scales: a 4-item, 0-10 pain severity scale (asking about pain in the morning, afternoon, evening, and with activity) and a 7-item pain interference scale asking how much pain interferes with more functional things like walking, normal work, and interactions with other people. If you're using a more detailed body diagram and are going to ask about medications during the history those sections can be removed to shorten the scale.	The pain severity scale (can either be reported as a sum /40 or an average /10) functions as any other pain intensity rating scale does, though the separation by time of day may be useful as you explore the patient's experiences further. Pain that is worse in the morning, eases through the day, then worse again in the evening may be more indicative of a peripheral mechanical or inflammatory driver than would be of constant severe pain. The interference subscale provides additional valuable information. We recently found it can be interpreted a single score or as 3 subscales: Physical Interference (walking, working, general activity), Affective Interference (social relationships, emotions, enjoyment of life), and Sleep Interference (single item). Patient responses on these items should then logically lead to more detailed evaluation if they appear troublesome.
Other reasonable options	There are several other scales and tools that generally fulfill the four criteria described earlier and could add richness to your go-to toolbox. These include tools we've created and published: the MultiDimensional Symptom Index (MSI) (Walton & Marsh 2018) and the Satisfaction and Recovery Index (Walton et al., 2015a). Other pain cognition tools could also be of value, though we suspect you will get enough of an overview from the tools already described and from sound clinical interview questions, though for those looking for others that also fulfill our 'go-to' criteria, the Pain Catastrophizing Scale (or any of its shortened versions), the Tampa Scale for Kinesiophobia, or the Fear-Avoidance Beliefs Questionnaire could be sound options, keeping in mind that the bulk of evidence for each is in the chronic low back pain field. The Patient-Specific Functional Scale also partly addresses the issue of personalized importance of items on tools. Co-morbidity scales, daily life stress scales, early life adversity scales, work-related demands scales, and any number of other more generic scales may also offer value for this purpose.	The multitude of tools that exist can provide additional information about domains of the patient's pain experience and you are encouraged to explore some of those.
To download these tools for your personal use in clinic, go to www.pirlresearch.com.		

information on meeting basic needs, physical and emotional resilience, connections with other people, sense of autonomy and spontaneity, and optimism for the future, in a metric we've termed 'importance-weighted health-related satisfaction'. The importance-weighting has an interesting mathematical effect, in that change on an item rated of high importance to the patient, leads to a larger overall change in scale score than does change on an item of low importance.

Another tool we recently created for this purpose is the MultiDimensional Symptom Index (MSI) (Walton & Marsh, 2018). The MSI includes 10 items and, similar to the SRI, two response scales. On the first pass, patients are asked to indicate how *often* they experience each of the 10 symptoms. On the second pass they indicate how much interference they experience as a result of each. The single tool takes about 90 seconds to complete (scoring requires an app or spreadsheet, that can be freely accessed for clinicians by contacting the authors) and provides very rich information: number of different symptoms experienced (out of 10), the mean frequency of those experiences (out of 3), the mean degree to which those symptoms interfere with function (out of 4), a composite frequency-by-interference score for each of the 10 different symptom types, and two subscales – one measuring more somatic complaints, and one measuring more non-somatic or central complaints. The individual symptom composite scores can also be used to create a radar plot of just the MSI. Thus a single, 90-second tool provides upwards of 17 or 18 different pieces of information. This is an example of a tool that we're stopping short of endorsing for routine use simply because the scoring requires a computer (not hard, but more time-consuming than those summed by hand). However, for those interested in deeper phenotyping we encourage you to check it out. These are further examples of other available PROs that would satisfy our four criteria for a 'go-to'

toolbox, but as of this writing our preferences remain those listed in Table 6.1.

Generic vs. region-specific tools

The final consideration here is where region-specific disability scales should come in. For example, in the neck region, the Neck Disability Index (NDI) is the most common; in the low back region, common scales include the Oswestry Disability Index (ODI) and the Roland-Morris Disability Questionnaire (RMDQ). For upper extremity problems, the Disabilities of the Arm, Shoulder and Hand (DASH) and the Upper Extremity Functional Index (UEFI) are popular options. The Lower Extremity Functional Scale (LEFS) or the Western Ontario McMaster Osteoarthritis Index (WOMAC) are widely used in studies of the lower extremities. The go-to tools described above have been intentionally chosen for their generic nature, but this would also be the time to provide a region-specific measure if needed. Some insurance or health policy-makers require specific tools be used to justify treatment, or ongoing care. While some clinics may have their own proprietary scales, many clinicians, like you, have their own favorite 'go-to' scales.

While generic tools allow comparison across patient populations (and you will soon learn how to identify troublesome scores), body-region-specific scales are meant only for people with a problem in that *region* of the body (hence the name). Some evidence suggests region-specific scales are more responsive to change as they are less likely to suffer from the irrelevant items problem that we described above for the BPI, but our initial work on the generic SRI found it to be just as responsive as the NDI for people with neck pain. Most of these scales are focused at the level of activity interference (walking, running, lifting, driving, etc.) though some also confound that by adding in symptom severity items, such as the NDI that includes items on pain intensity and headache severity/frequency amongst the other functional items. These scales however do have other values – for example, the NDI has been shown to be a useful prognostic indicator when trying to identify those people at high risk of chronic pain, and all have shown evidence for being responsive to change in patient status so can be quite useful as 'tracking tools' over time. However, the nature of the questions are not as useful as the other tools described here for creating a profile of your patient's pain experience, nor do they offer as much guidance towards specific treatment options; that is, while a patient may indicate they are having a problem with driving or lifting, there's little that can be gleaned from that regarding the mechanisms to explain *why* they're having that trouble. So, while region-specific scales are valuable and, in most cases, can be captured at a patient's first visit as a baseline to follow over time, they are considered a fringe inclusion in your go-to toolbox from the APT perspective as they offer little guidance for triangulation or creating a radar plot.

Summary

Having tools in your 'go-to toolbox' that are brief, generic, provide rich information, and are adequately valid is a great place to start with all patients presenting with pain, and may be a good first step into the use of routine outcome measures for those who don't already use them. The tools we've described here are useful for starting to phenotype your patient, though as we've mentioned, they're less valuable for tracking change in patient status over time. While the BPI is the most useful for this, the responsiveness of most body diagrams and the BIPQ are less established.

For this, one additional tool such as a region-specific functional measure that you may already be required to use, or a patient-centric tool like PSFS, COPM or SRI, would be a valuable addition as a 'tracking tool'. For subsequent visits, your tracking tool can be used to routinely track change over time

or effectiveness of your intervention, while your go-to toolbox may only need to be used again if you want to recreate that patient's profile on the radar plot as part of a comprehensive re-assessment.

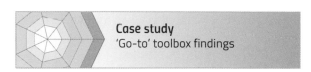

Case study
'Go-to' toolbox findings

Sean Terwilliger is 38 years old, and married with two children aged 8 and 10. He is an Executive Assistant for an international import/export company. He was involved in a motor vehicle collision in which the car he was in was hit from behind while at a traffic light one week ago. He was a belted front-seat passenger. Having a busy life and being the primary breadwinner for his household, he carried on with his normal activities for the next two days. On the third day following the crash he awoke with severe neck stiffness and a supra-orbital left-sided headache. He tried to work but had to leave half way through the day to visit his family doctor. His doctor diagnosed him with 'whiplash' and prescribed NSAIDs before referring him on.

When you see Sean, he is clearly uncomfortable, tending to support his neck with his hand during the interview. He rates his current pain at 7/10, which has not changed much over the past two days. Sean reports that he is, for the most part, healthy. He regularly visits the gym 3-4 times per week for weight-training and general fitness. He played high-school football and enjoys cycling for recreation. He reports having had a few 'zingers' during high-school football and has fractured his collar-bone falling from his bicycle that causes some occasional shoulder stiffness but nothing major. He reports recurrent bouts of neck and headache pain in the past that he attributes to his previous athletic endeavors and his current job where he spends 'a lot' of time in front of a computer and traveling. He frequently receives treatments from a chiropractor and massage therapist which seem to provide some temporary relief.

Sean presents with left-sided neck pain that occasionally radiates into his left arm as far as the elbow and affects the back of his head (see body diagram, Fig. 6.1). He states his vision feels a bit 'off' and this has affected his reading of papers and working on his computer, as his eyes become fatigued quickly.

This also tends to increase his headache that he rates as a 4/10 while reading and an 8/10 when moving his neck. He describes difficulty driving since the event and finds that it is difficult to concentrate when attending to his peripheral vision. He denies numbness/tingling into his upper or lower extremities.

Brief Pain Inventory findings

Pain severity (left neck and head):
- Worst = 8/10
- Least = 3/10
- Average = 7/10
- Right now = 7/10

Pain interference:
- Total = 35/70 (moderate interference, higher number worse)
- Physical interference = 12/30
- Affective interference – 18/30
- Sleep interference = 5/10

Body diagram

Sean's completed body diagram is shown in Figure 6.1.

Interpretation

From just the background and these tools, we can extract considerable information:
- Recent acute traumatic mechanism of injury (nociceptive)
- Unilateral left-sided symptoms that increase with movement (nociceptive)
- Difficulty concentrating, eye strain, attending to peripheral vision (sensorimotor, maybe central nociplastic)
- Higher stress job, primary income earner (socioenvironmental)
- No numbness/tingling, no radiation beyond the elbow (negative neuropathic)
- Pain severity high but fluctuates (slightly more nociceptive than central, but hard to say)
- More affective than physical pain-related interference, moderate sleep interference (some evidence for emotional)

Table 6.2	Brief Illness Perceptions Questionnaire (BIPQ)	
1	Negative effect on life	6
2	Expected duration	4
3	*Sense of control*	3
4	*Belief in treatment*	5
5	Number of symptoms	5
6	Severity of symptoms	8
7	Level of concern	7
8	*Understanding of the condition*	5
9	Sense of fragility/risk of injury	8
10	Negative effect on emotions	8

All BIPQ items are scored out of 10. For items 1, 2, 5, 6, 7, 9, and 10, a higher number would indicate a more distressing experience/more threatening appraisal of the symptoms. For items 3, 4, and 8 (italics), a higher number indicates a less distressing experience/less threatening appraisal of the symptoms. Generally speaking, scores ≥ 7/10 (for the negatively oriented items) or ≤3/10 (for the positively oriented items) are worth exploring further. Collectively, Sean's scores indicate that he is appraising the symptoms as quite threatening or distressing (see for example Walton et al., 2015b).

- Body diagram indicates symptoms in a definable area (nociceptive)
- BIPQ (Table 6.2) indicates generally high distress/threat value assigned to the symptoms, high sense of fragility and low sense of control (cognitive and emotional)

While more information is needed for triangulation, and it is too early to have strong confidence in any one driver, we can start to shape Sean's radar plot with just this rich information (Fig. 6.2).

On the diagrams below, please indicate the areas in which you are currently feeling symptoms.

1 Shade (color) the areas in which you are feeling pain.

2 Circle in the areas in which you are feeling tingling, prickling or burning.

3 Place an 'N' near the areas where you are feeling numbness, heaviness or other sensations.

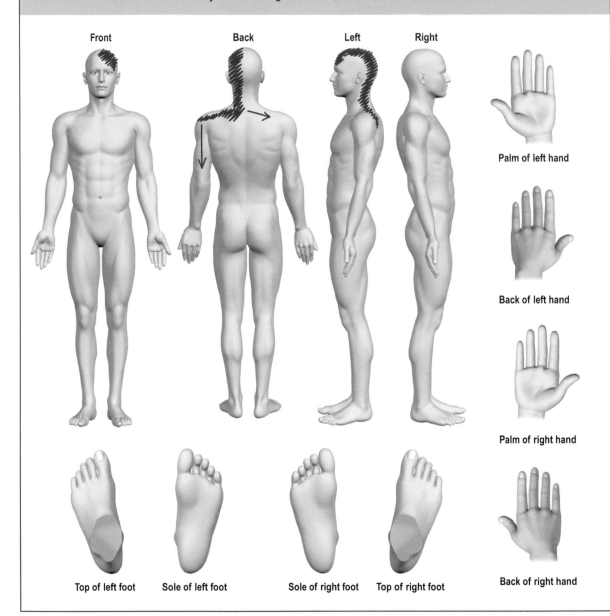

Figure 6.1
Sean's completed body diagram.

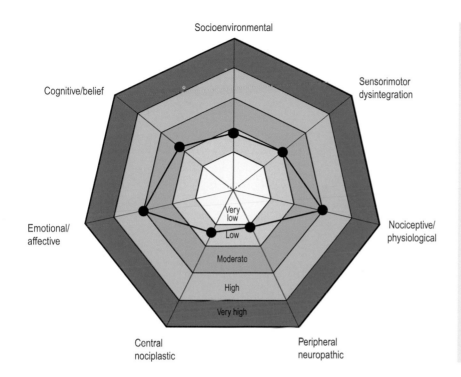

Figure 6.2
The radar plot begins to take shape, based on the information gleaned from Sean's history and the 'go-to' toolbox findings. We will revisit Sean's radar plot in subsequent chapters.

References

Barney, C. C., Stibb, S. M., Merbler, A. M., et al., 2018. Psychometric properties of the Brief Pain Inventory modified for proxy report of pain interference in children with cerebral palsy with and without cognitive impairment. *Pain Reports* 3 (4):e666.

Broadbent, E., Petrie, K.J., Main, J., et al., 2006. The Brief Illness Perception Questionnaire. *Journal of Psychosomatic Research* 60:631–7.

Cleeland, C. S., Ryan, K. M., 1994. Pain assessment: global use of the Brief Pain Inventory. *Annals of the Academy of Medicine, Singapore* 23 (2):129–38.

Darnall, B. D., Sazie, E., 2012. Pain characteristics and pain catastrophizing in incarcerated women with chronic pain. *Journal of Health Care for the Poor and Underserved* 23 (2):543–56.

Law, M., Baptiste, S., McColl, M., et al., 1990. The Canadian Occupational Performance Measure: an outcome measure for occupational therapy. *Canadian Journal of Occupational Therapy* 57 (2):82–7.

Walton, D. M., Balsor, B., Etruw, E., 2012. Exploring the causes of neck pain and disability as perceived by those who experience the condition: a mixed-methods study. *ISRN Rehabilitation* 2012, Article ID 971328, 7 pages. https://doi.org/10.5402/2012/971328.

Walton, D. M., Macdermid, J. C., Taylor, T., et al., 2013. What does 'recovery' mean to people with neck pain? Results of a descriptive thematic analysis. *The Open Orthopaedics Journal* 7:420–7.

Walton, D. M., MacDermid , J. C., Pulickal, M., et al., 2014. Development and initial validation of the Satisfaction and Recovery Index (SRI) for measurement of recovery from musculoskeletal trauma. *The Open Orthopaedics Journal* 8:316–25.

Walton, D. M., 2015. Making (common) sense of outcome measures. *Manual Therapy* 20 (6):723–6.

Walton, D., MacDermid, J., Pulickal, M., et al., 2015a. The Satisfaction and Recovery Index as a new generic measure of health-related satisfaction: development and preliminary validation. *Physiotherapy* 101 (Suppl 1):e1596.

Walton, D. M., Lefebvre, A., Reynolds, D., 2015b. The Brief Illness Perceptions Questionnaire identifies 3 classes of people seeking rehabilitation for mechanical neck pain. *Manual Therapy* 20 (3):420–6.

Walton, D. M., Putos, J., Beattie, T., et al., 2016. Confirmatory factor analysis of 2 versions of the Brief Pain Inventory in an ambulatory population indicates that sleep interference should be interpreted separately. *Scandinavian Journal of Pain* 12: 110–6.

Walton, D. M., Marsh, J., 2018. The Multidimensional Symptom Index: A new patient-reported outcome for pain phenotyping, prognosis and treatment decisions. *European Journal of Pain* 22 (7):1351–61.

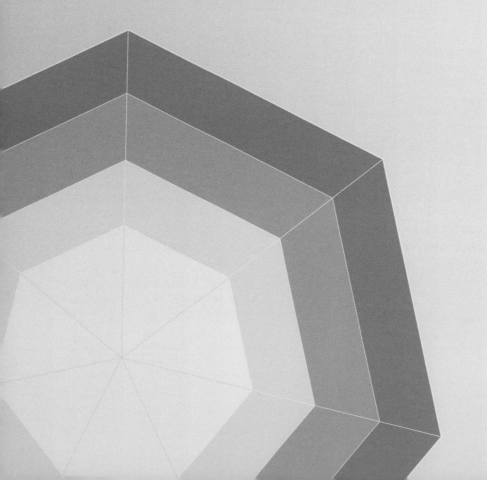

7

The Physiological Nociceptive Domain

The seven radar plot domains

Having now provided the foundational information on the experience and reporting of pain, the assess-predict-treat clinical reasoning framework, the use of radar plots and triangulation for making sense of information, and the idea of a go-to-toolbox, we now turn to deeper exploration of each of the seven points on the radar plot. Each of the chapters in this second section of the book are arranged similarly, starting with a description of the domain and proposed mechanisms, key clinical signs, a list of potential tools/techniques for identifying it, and guidance on treatment decisions when that domain is deemed to be a strong driver of the pain experience. At the end of each chapter we provide additional information about that domain for the case of Sean Terwilliger, introduced in Chapter 6. Additional cases with more ambiguous information are provided in the final chapter for readers to practice their new skills in pain assessment, interpretation, and phenotyping.

Proposed mechanisms of the physiological nociceptive domain

A pain experience with strong peripheral nociceptive input, sometimes referred to as a 'physiological' driver, is one that receives input starting from the end organ (free nerve ending) of a high-threshold nerve, often of the A-delta or C polymodal class. These nociceptive afferent fibers appear to express receptors on their free nerve endings capable of transducing (turning one type of stimulus into an electric signal) noxious or potentially noxious-level stimuli of either a mechanical (e.g. pressure, stretch), thermal (e.g. strong heat or cold), or chemical (e.g. inflammatory mediators such as bradykinins, prostaglandins or hydrogen ions) nature. Pain from acute injuries like an ankle sprain, a superficial burn, or a paper cut probably have a strong nociceptive driver, though keep in mind that pain is never *only* a result of one type of input, and that tissue damage is neither necessary nor sufficient for any one individual's highly personal experience of pain.

Several intracellular signaling pathways have been described for different types of stimuli that may start with activation of transient receptor potential (TRP) voltage-gated channels, chemically (e.g. calcium) gated channels, mechanically gated channels, or sodium voltage-gated (Nav1) channels, among others (Fig. 7.1). The cyclooxygenase-2 (COX-2) pathway is one with which some readers may be familiar, having been the target of the ill-fated, yet ubiquitous for a time, Merck analgesic drug Vioxx (rofecoxib) that was unceremoniously pulled from the market due to risk of cardiovascular side effects in 2004 (Krumholz et al., 2007). The other COX inhibitors now bear an FDA-mandated 'black box warning' of cardiovascular (CV) and gastrointestinal (GI) risks. In fact, the American Heart Association warns that patients with a prior history of or at high risk of CV disease should limit their use of COX-2 inhibitors for their pain relief, and in the case of no appropriate alternative, only the lowest dose and shortest duration should be considered (Antman et al., 2007). In other words, while knowing the pathway from injury to pain is valuable, we should always exercise caution when attempting to interfere.

The consistent characteristic of the mechanism of action in pain of primarily nociceptive origin is that an adequately strong stimulation (one at the intensity to cause or possibly cause peripheral tissue damage) opens channels in the nerve cell membrane leading to depolarization of the cell. This depolarization starts the process of a rapid shift of ions between the intra- and extracellular space, and if of adequate threshold, an action potential 'spikes', propagating across membrane ion channels from the periphery to the central nervous system (CNS). It is at the CNS, in the dorsal horn of the spinal cord, that the first order peripheral nerves synapse with second order neurons commonly referred to as *nociceptive specific* (NS) or *wide dynamic range* (WDR) neurons. These second order neurons project cranially to the thalamus and other brain regions for integration, perception, interpretation, and action. Like any signal coming from the periphery, it will be subject to modification along its path including at the terminal synapses of the primary peripheral afferent in the dorsal horn, or at any of the relay stations in the brain. There appear to be several strong influences on the signal that can lead to its up- or down-regulation

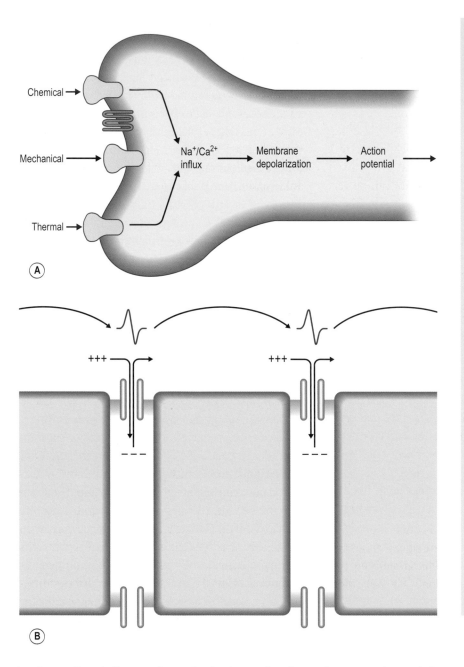

Figure 7.1
(**A**) Diagrammatic representation of transduction of chemical, mechanical or thermal stimuli into action potentials through specific membrane channels. Intense stimuli are enough to 'open the gates' in the nerve membrane allowing the rapid influx of positive ions (calcium and sodium) leading to depolarization of the normally polarized membrane and creation of a new action potential. (**B**) The action potential is propagated along the nerve membranes through junctions in the myelin sheath (Nodes of Ranvier), as voltage-gated channels allow the influx of positive (sodium) and outflux of negative (chloride) ions. After their action potential passes, membrane pumps actively work to re-establish the potential difference across the membrane to prepare the cell for the next wave of impulses.

by descending influence from the brain, or by the multiple other players that reside in the central nervous system such as interneurons and immunoreactive glial cells. These findings have led experts in the field to opine that the message reaching the brain for interpretation and the resulting conscious experience should not be considered an accurate reflection of what exactly is happening out in the periphery; rather it is a complex, coordinated, interaction between the peripheral and central nervous systems that may bear little resemblance to what is actually happening in the tissues. Examples of the non-linear nature of this complex phenomenon include stories of shark attacks wherein victims often describe the sensation as a 'bump' or a 'jiggle' rather than excruciating pain, when tissue damage has clearly occurred. Other stories, of people who have been shot, stabbed (or otherwise injured), without being consciously aware of it are examples of how, even in the context of a primary nociceptive driver, the actual *experience* can be very different from what is happening in the tissues. Clearly the signal can be modified, amplified, suppressed, or completely inhibited based on any number of other influences on, and in, the brain.

While it has been well established that there is not a direct one-to-one relationship between the magnitude of tissue damage and the magnitude of pain experienced or expressed, many pain experiences can still trace their origins back to an initiating tissue damage event with subsequent, and expected, peripheral nociceptive input. As stated above, this 'physiological' process is driven by the action potential originating at the level of a peripheral receptor on an end organ, traveling *orthodromically* ('the correct direction down a path') towards the spinal cord and ultimately to the brain. This naming method can be useful when it comes to distinguishing physiological from non-physiological peripheral nerve activity, which is often the case in neuropathic pain conditions (where signals arise mid-nerve and travel both *ortho-* and *antidromically*, that latter meaning 'the wrong direction') (Fig. 7.2). (More on antidromic conduction in Chapter 8).

Once it reaches the brain, input from the periphery is then scrutinized and interpreted in light of other information to which the brain has access, such as the context in which the experience is occurring, the emotional state of the person (prior to, during, and after the 'injury'), past experiences with similar sensations, and a host of other information, to determine if the most appropriate 'output' of the system should be pain or something else. This makes sense in light of evolutionary theory around pain as part of the diverse protective mechanisms intended to promote; it may not be advantageous to scream and hop around in pain when trying to escape a saber-tooth tiger. Clearly, such an explanation helps reinforce that pain is highly individual and each person has their own experience with it, despite a similar mechanism for how the injury (e.g. an ankle sprain) and pain came to be.

It's important to remember that pain is not the *only* possible outcome of your brain being alerted to, and becoming aware of, tissue damage – motor (escape), autonomic (fight/flight/freeze), immune (fight infection), or in some cases even a paradoxical euphoria could all be alternative outputs. The ability to facilitate or suppress the experience of pain is especially useful if the brain believes that a better survival strategy given the circumstances is not to yell 'ouch' or limp around, but perhaps to swim or run quickly away from whatever is causing the damage, or to activate your innate immune system to fend off infection.

Previous pain scholars have created models or frameworks from which to understand the imperfect relationship between nociceptive input and the pain output. Melzack's Neuromatrix Model (Fig. 7.3) posits that pain is the most likely output only when the results of scrutinizing the input in terms of its sensory-discriminative characteristics (Where is it coming from? How intense is it?), its cognitive-evaluative characteristics (What happened the last time I felt this? What does it mean?), and its motivational-affective components (How does it make me feel? Does it make me want to escape?) all indicate actual or potential damage. Figure 7.4 represents Gifford's Mature Organism Model, which offers a similar conceptualization of the experience of pain, proposing a process through which the brain samples all of its available information, internally, externally,

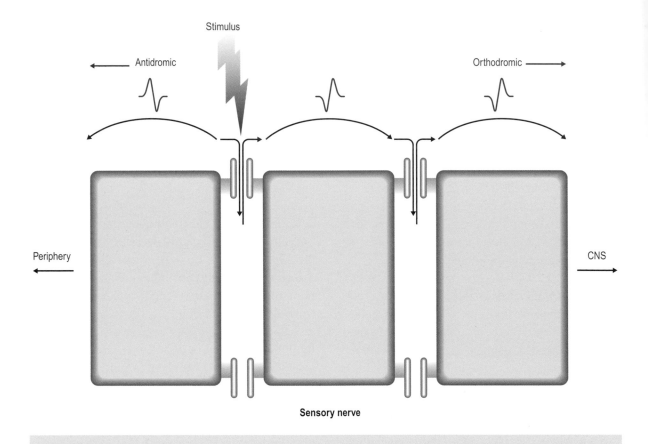

Figure 7.2
Diagrammatic representation of orthodromic and antidromic action potential propagation. This being a sensory afferent, 'normal' direction of propagation is back towards the central nervous system (spinal cord and brain). Of course, nerve membranes have no valves (unlike veins) so depolarization is free to spread in all directions across the membrane. In this case, a stimulus applied in the mid-portion of the nerve will also travel antidromically, which in this case would be out towards the periphery. If this were instead a motor efferent, the relative directions of ortho/antidromic propagation would be in the opposite directions. We will discuss the impacts of this type of non-physiological propagation in Chapter 8.

and archived, to attempt to answer the question: how dangerous is this *really*? (Gifford, 1998).

Astute readers will recognize that the concept of a purely mechanical or 'physiological' pain in the absence of cognitions, emotions, and contextual information is not in keeping with our current knowledge of pain science – rather all such inputs need to indicate threat or harm for the person to experience or express what most of us would consider pain (Box 7.1) A pain experience driven *primarily* by a nociceptive or physiological driver can be identified most easily by a patient presentation consistent with a mechanical, inflammatory, or thermal stimulus, but again we remind readers that such stimuli in isolation are neither adequate nor sufficient to lead to a pain experience, nor should the magnitude of damage be taken as 'proof' that a patient is or is not in pain, or is behaving in a way that

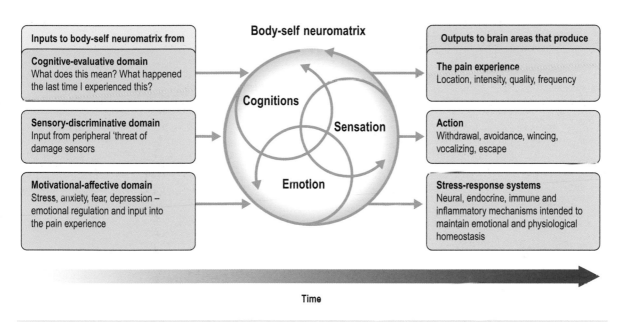

Figure 7.3
An adapted version of the Neuromatrix Model of pain as described by Melzack (1999). Inputs into the body-self neuromatrix include sensory, cognitive, and affective influences. Outputs in response to potential threat include pain, action systems, and stress-regulation systems. Note that in this model the entire process is internal to the person, there is no indication of social or contextual influence. (Adapted from Melzack, R., 1999. From the gate to the neuromatrix. *Pain* Suppl 6:S121–6.)

'adequately' and 'appropriately' aligns with the intensity of that pain. Where and when a relatively strong nociceptive/physiological driver appears to exist, clinical findings should start to point to signs that a nociceptive driver is influencing the clinical course; more so than other domains detailed in the radar plot. This type of pain profile is most likely to be amenable to traditional and conservative pain management techniques such as non-steroidal anti-inflammatory drugs, tissue unloading techniques, bracing, splinting, thermal or electrotherapeutic modalities, or specific exercise (see below for intervention strategies).

Distinguishing features

The most useful distinguishing feature of pain with a strong physiologic nociceptive driver is a consistent association between the behavior of the symptoms and the stimulus. So if the aggravating stimulus is mechanical (e.g. stretch or compression), then clinicians should be able to identify specific movements that consistently aggravate the pain experience (increase the pain) and others that consistently relieve it. In this way, both aggravation and relief are predictable, and occur in a way that is in keeping with current anatomical and biomechanical knowledge. This is not to say the pain experience doesn't fluctuate throughout the day – indeed it may be more intense early in the morning, after long periods of inactivity, or later in the evening, but even these are usually consistent patterns that the patient will describe and are typical of a 'normal' physiological (e.g. body healing itself) response to injury.

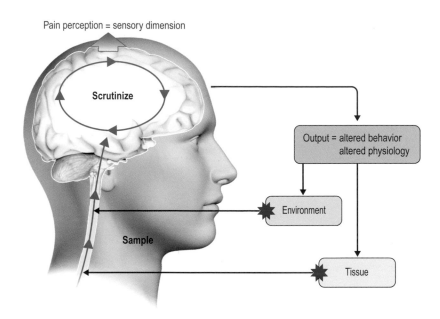

Figure 7.4
An adapted version of Gifford's Mature Organism Model (1998). Similar to the Neuromatrix Model, the MOM proposes multiple inputs into the cortex that are scrutinized, and if a determination of 'current or potential threat or harm' is made, then pain, altered behavior and altered physiological processes are the result. This model does incorporate external environment with internal processes, though focuses largely on tissue-based inputs to initiate the process. (Adapted with permission from Gifford, L., 1998. Pain, the tissues and the nervous system: A conceptual model. Physiotherapy 84 (1):27–36. Copyright © 1998 Chartered Society of Physiotherapy. Published by Elsevier Ltd.)

Think again of the acute ankle sprain. We've all likely 'rolled' an ankle playing organized sport, or while walking through the garden or on uneven terrain. The experience, which is usually short-lived, is not long forgotten. The feeling of our ankle rolling 'over itself' with an immediate feeling of fear that something bad just happened, followed by that intense burst of pain, confirming that something potentially bad has indeed just happened. Over the next few days we are reminded of the injury as just about every movement aggravates our ankle, which is now swollen, and perhaps a bit 'black and blue' in color. Soon, however, we recognize that specific positions or gentle movements consistently relieve the acute pain, which is now giving rise to even more movement, less inflammation, and markedly fewer

Box 7.1 What is pain?

Intense unpleasant sensations
Negative emotions
Behaviors intended to reduce or avoid further damage and/or signal to others that help is needed

visual reminders of bruising. In short, we soon begin to move our ankle, put a bit of weight on it and gain the confidence that tissue healing is occurring. While our ankle may never be the same as it was before the injury, we are on our way to regaining pain-free movement. The key indicator here is the consistency of the behavior of the pain.

Movement-based analyses are therefore useful for discriminating nociceptive pain drivers from others on the plot. If, for example, the anterior talofibular ligament (ATFL) is a likely culprit, you would expect not only point tenderness on palpation, but also a consistent pattern of pain reproduction wherein pain worsens when the ankle is plantarflexed and inverted (position of tension of the ATFL), and relieved when the tension is released. To move to another body region, if a cervical facet (zygapophyseal) joint is the likely culprit of a person's neck pain, perhaps as a result of pathological compression of the innervated intra- or periarticular structures, then you may expect pain consistently worsens in a position of maximum compression (extension, ipsilateral side bend and rotation) and is eased with the opposite movement (flexion, contralateral side bend and rotation) (Fig. 7.5). Assuming the tissue culprit is adequately superficial, local tenderness on palpation, in the absence of widespread tenderness, may be another distinguishing characteristic of facet-mediated pain (Fig. 7.6A&B). A special caveat is required here though, in that particularly with inflammatory drivers, a zone of *secondary hyperalgesia* may be identifiable around the primary area of tissue damage. This secondary hyperalgesia zone may display slightly odd characteristics, including sensory allodynia (heightened unpleasant experience in response to light brushing), hypoesthesia (reduced tactile acuity, numbness) or other things that would otherwise suggest a neuropathic pain driver. The diagnostic criteria for neuropathy are now fairly clear and are discussed in the next section. For the purposes of this driver, secondary hyperalgesia may be identified, but the consistent pain behavior patterns in response to movement or palpation remain the hallmark criteria for this nociceptive domain.

Diagnostic imaging

This is also the type of driver for which diagnostic imaging may be most useful, and this is worth some discussion. While it is true that not all abnormalities on imaging are associated with pain, and that pain can be present in the absence of observable lesions, when a lesion is clearly present on imaging and is logically consistent with the pain experiences of

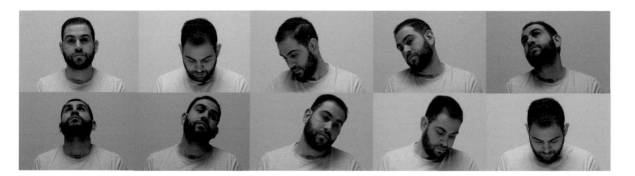

Figure 7.5
An example of a clinical test for identifying consistent signs of cervical nociceptive input. *Cervical circumduction* involves the patient 'rolling' their head in as large a circle as they can around their shoulders and upper back until returning to the start position. In the case of an articular compression problem, the patient can get 'stuck' or move particularly slowly or cautiously, or indicate pain, in one of the posterior right or left quadrants. Importantly, this experience of pain should be similar regardless of whether they start by rolling their head to the left or to the right.

the patient, this would seem a strong indication of a nociceptive physiological driver. Our position is that, despite some occasionally vociferous commentary to the contrary, the presence of pathology in some people with spinal or bodily pain should not be dismissed as a normal variant on grounds they are also present in some people without these conditions. A potential risk of 'forgetting' a biological component of pain is the stifling of important research that aims to better understand the contribution of local pathology and the generation, if not maintenance, of pain. We argue that high quality research (especially those using and combining new technologies) investigating the potential biological contributors to a patient's pain experience form an important part of this line of inquiry. Without a better mechanistic understanding of the many biological contributors, it is likely the personal, societal, and economic burden of pain will remain unchanged, enormous, and not 'uncomplicated'.

We largely agree with the recommendations to avoid routine, non-indicated imaging for spinal pain, and we further endorse that routine imaging should not be conducted once the patient has been medically screened and determined to not have serious pathology. However, we believe this whole discourse and resulting actions to reduce unwarranted imaging and diagnostic tests risk producing a message that all imaging and diagnostic tests are unnecessary, and they should not be performed. In purest terms, we argue some of the movements against imaging or diagnostic tests have been somewhat premature, as the research and those who endorse it should realize they are stuck in something of a logical loop. If pain is complex and multifactorial, then why should we think any single variable, including dodgy-looking joint surfaces on imaging, should be able to independently explain significant variance in pain? What is more likely to come to light eventually is that those dodgy joints, in a person with the right (or wrong, depending on

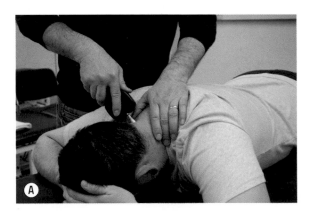 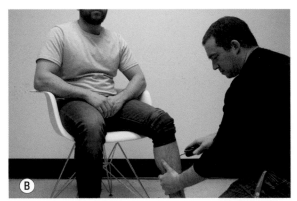

Figure 7.6
A quantitative method for testing local mechanical hyperalgesia. (**A**) An algometer (force transducer) with a 1cm² rubber tip is pushed into the tissue over the painful area increasing at a rate of 5 N/s until the patient indicates that the sensation has changed from pressure to pain. This is called the 'pressure pain detection threshold' (PPDT), and evidence for a nociceptive driver is provided when local hyperalgesia is present but not widespread hyperalgesia. There are normative data tables available for some body regions, and a free app can be downloaded from http://www.pirlresearch.com/clinician-resources. Note that when testing local PPDT for the neck, we often also test an anatomically distinct region. In this case, the tibialis anterior (**B**), for which we also offer free normative data information, available from the same link.

your perspective) combination of genetics, life experiences, previous medical history, prior exposures to trauma, stress, and lifestyle may be quite important for understanding a person's pain experience. There's got to be some reason why, in some people, cutting out a 'nasty looking' femoral condyle and tibial plateau and replacing it with shiny aftermarket parts dramatically reduces knee pain. Joint arthroplasty is not universally effective of course, nor is it effective to the same degree in those who get relief. In some people things go from bad to worse following the surgery despite post-operative images suggesting 'nothing is wrong' and that the replacement part looks to be secure. Perhaps (if we are to be a bit contentious) the mechanism driving relief in those who have successful surgery is purely placebo. Regardless, this is all part of the same point: it is folly to try and reduce the experience of pain to any single factor, whether that be cognition, biomechanics, structural pathology on imaging, or culture. A more compelling question in our minds coming from those studies showing similar proportions of structural pathology in those without pain would be: what factors are protective against pain in the asymptomatic group, or what are the vulnerabilities present in the symptomatic group? We suspect there are many more chapters to be written in this story as research and practice continue to evolve.

Suggested evidence for triangulation

In every chapter we will provide a table like the one below describing potential evidence for triangulating each domain as a potential driver of the pain experience, along with the shift in the likelihood (the magnitude that the point on the radar plot changes) in response to a positive or negative result. These are again quite intentionally qualitative in nature, and you will likely be hard-pressed to find concrete empirical evidence to support many of these. Rather, what you are getting is the collective experience, and we daresay a touch of wisdom, from a couple of people who have spent considerable time in the field of musculoskeletal pain. Due to the somewhat novel nature of the domains on our plot, even the diagnostic accuracy (shift in likelihood) is largely opinion-based as many such signs and symptoms have not been explored in the context of the seven radar plot domains.

With that in mind, here is your first table.

Suggested evidence for triangulation: nociceptive domain		
Test domains	**Findings**	**Shift in likelihood**
Symptom behavior	Pain, reduced mobility, and/or swelling are primary complaints	++
	Localized complaints with a clear epicenter, but may be radiation in a definable distribution (dermatome, sclerotome, or peripheral innervation region)	+
	Representative qualities are sharp, stabbing, dull, or achy	+
	Pain and/or stiffness may be worse on waking in the morning, after periods of immobility, or in the evening	+
	Movement generally relieves pain and stiffness	++
	Symptoms are amenable to simple analgesics or NSAIDs	++
	Patient history is consistent with either a traumatic or insidious non-neuropathic mechanism that could have logically led to the clinical presentation	+

continued—

	Suggested evidence for triangulation: nociceptive domain *continued*	

Test domains	Findings	Shift in likelihood
Palpation	Local hyperalgesia	+
	Consistent reproduction of pain on palpation	+
	Palpable lesion or defect	++
	No allodynia	+
Quantitative sensory testing	Local mechanical sensitivity only, no widespread hyperalgesia	++
	Local thermal hypersensitivity *may* be present but only in a defined region (think: sunburn)	+
	Two-point discrimination and light touch are intact	+
	Conditioned pain modulation functions well	++
Sensorimotor testing	In purest terms, when pain is *primarily* being driven by nociceptive input and proprioceptive input is spared, there should be no signs of sensorimotor dysfunction. We note however that it is rare for tissue to be damaged while proprioception is spared, so the two phenomena often co-occur.	+
Mechanical testing	Pain is consistently reproduced with a characteristic mechanical pattern of movement (e.g. stretch or compression quadrants)	+++
	Manual muscle testing or selective tissue tension testing identify impairments that could logically be causing, or are a result of, a peripheral lesion	+
Cognitions	No definable pattern	+
Emotions	No definable pattern	+
Socioenvironmental	No definable pattern	+
Pathology	Imaging may identify a lesion (e.g. tear, bulge, or fracture) or pathological process (e.g. degeneration) that could logically give rise to the clinical complaints	++

+, small shift in likelihood that the domain in question is a strong driver; ++, moderate shift in likelihood; +++, strong shift in likelihood.

Prognostic value

Of the radar plot domains, a profile suggesting a strong nociceptive driver in the absence of other strong drivers probably offers the least information in terms of expected natural or clinical course. We note that it is uncommon to find a 'clean' nociceptive profile without contributions from other domains (e.g. cognitions, emotions, socioenvironmental context), especially as the pain experience persists. As such, there are few (though some) prognostic studies that have adequately explored signs that would be in the nociceptive/physiological domain that predict outcome. Rather, most findings from research arise from studies that attempted to recruit a homogenous group of patients to limit confounders arising from the messiness of being human, meaning that those researchers do their best to avoid people with strong emotional or sensorimotor drivers, though such people are rarely seen in clinical practice.

It is however noteworthy, that in the acute pain condition, it is possible to see a strong nociceptive profile, and of the anticipated recovery trajectories, these are the patients most likely to follow the rapid recovery trajectory. This statement is based on the existing prognostic evidence suggesting cognitive and emotional influences, context, and sensory processing disorders are stronger predictors of outcome than are traditional biomechanical or inflammatory factors. As such this statement is more about the *lack* of other poor prognostic factors rather than some protective effect offered by nociceptive drivers. Where these drivers have been explored, they have mostly not proven to be strong prognostic factors. We've explored the use of pressure pain detection threshold and found that local sensitivity in the absence of widespread sensory changes do little to predict who gets better and who does not. One of the more rigorous evaluations of this domain comes from Helge Kasch and colleagues, who created a risk stratification paradigm that includes, amongst a host of other variables from different domains, restricted range of motion in the cervical spine to identify those at greatest risk of non-recovery from whiplash (Kasch et al., 2011). In their risk protocol, significantly restricted range of motion in multiple planes is one of the signs on which to base a poor prognosis. Even here however, it would be hard to say with confidence that restricted range is not due to something else, like fear avoidance or sensorimotor integration problems and dizziness, unless the pattern of restriction was, as described earlier, consistent and showed a pattern that made sense.

Overall, in the case of high or very high confidence in an acute nociceptive profile without strong contributions from other drivers, clinicians can most confidently predict rapid recovery over a period of 6 to 12 weeks for most musculoskeletal conditions with minimal intervention.

Intervention strategies

In the acute post-injury phase, patients with a strong nociceptive profile are probably best suited to existing clinical practice guidelines or protocols that endorse advice, education, and reassurance. Advice should focus on simple pain management strategies to be used in the short term such as over-the-counter analgesics, ice, bracing or splinting, or if needed, rest or unloading techniques such as crutches. Education should focus on the nature of the injury, the expected time to recovery, and signs to watch for that would suggest recovery is not occurring as expected or that further workup may be needed. Reassurance should come in the form of explaining to the patient that based on their presentation and the results of your assessment there are no obvious signs to suggest recovery will not occur as expected for the condition and that lingering problems are unlikely.

Physical interventions in the acute phase should focus on tissue unloading or support if needed, active movement of the injured area within reasonable pain limits, and the appropriate use of medications or thermal modalities. It is unlikely that someone with an acute nociceptive profile will have suddenly experienced loss of muscle mass or loss of tissue length that would justify the initiation of a new, vigorous strengthening or stretching program, and it is possible that doing so may retard recovery as much as complete rest and immobilization. As a general rule, advice to 'maintain your usual routine as best you can' is sound for this type of presentation, be it low back pain, an acute ankle sprain, or a wry neck.

As pain persists, the balance of domains driving the experience tends to shift from nociceptive towards more central nociplastic and cognitive or emotional domains. As such, 'biomechanically' focused interventions may become lower priority or in some cases even contraindicated. This is especially true if a patient has become overly reliant on passive or manual therapies, or in the presence of exercise-induced hyperalgesia (a phenomenon that will be discussed in Chapter 9), even exercise may not be an appropriate first-line intervention. While not terribly helpful, it should be noted that evidence to support many interventions for chronic pain of nociceptive or other origin, especially when provided in isolation, is very weak. Where some optimism can be found is in the multimodal or interdisciplinary strategies. If a strong nociceptive driver is identified in a person with chronic pain, evidence from neck and low back pain does provide some support for a combination therapy approach that includes appropriate medication, manual therapies, exercise, and education (though the latter is more appropriate with a strong cognitive driver). There are few 'passive' therapeutic modalities that have shown benefit for patients with chronic pain, though acupuncture/dry needling may offer some benefit over placebo in the right patient, and transcutaneous electrical nerve stimulation (TENS) may similarly offer some degree of benefit. As will be stated throughout this book, *nothing works for everyone, but everything will work for someone.* Therefore, the consistent challenge for the clinician is to match the right treatment to the right person at the right time, which is why we focus so strongly on sound assessment and prognosis in the APT framework.

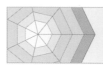

Case study
Physiological/nociceptive domain findings

Clinical examination

On observation of Sean, he is clearly guarded in his movements even when sitting at rest.

Clinical neurological findings (sensation and reflexes) are largely normal. Myotomal (isometric muscle strength) testing is inconclusive as most resisted movements of the neck and shoulder girdle are described as painful, but more distal testing is considered within normal limits.

Active movements reveal that he is restricted in his movements and his pain increases when moving in all directions, though more so in a consistent fashion when you ask him to extend and side-flex his neck left, or when you ask him to flex and side-flex right. Both lead to increases in posterior left-sided neck pain, and flexion increases his left-sided headache.

When testing mechanical pressure pain detection threshold of the posterior neck (upper trapezius muscles) with an algometer, he shows a very low threshold on the left and a moderately low threshold on the right. When testing over the tibialis anterior (anterior shin) muscles as a distal comparator, your findings indicate normal mechanical pain thresholds there (no signs of widespread hypersensitivity).

Passive mechanical/segmental testing is inconclusive owing to increased muscle tone/guarding.

Going back to our radar plot (Fig. 7.7), these results appear to lend more support to a nociceptive/physiological driver than to a central nociplastic driver. There is considerable evidence of a strong nociceptive driver now, so we're going to bump that point up a bit further on the plot.

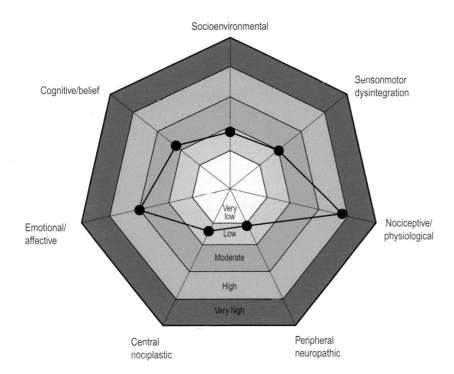

Socioenvironmental

Sensorimotor
dysintegration

Cognitive/belief

Nociceptive/
physiological

Emotional/
affective

Very
low

Low

Moderate

High

Very high

Central
nociplastic

Peripheral
neuropathic

Figure 7.7
Sean's radar plot continues
to take shape. Based on the
physiological/nociceptive
domain findings, this driver
has been moved to 'high'
probability.

References

Antman, E. M., Bennett, J. S., Daugherty, A., et al., 2007. Use of nonsteroidal anti-inflammatory drugs: an update for clinicians. A Scientific Statement from the American Heart Association. *Circulation* 115 (12):1634–42.

Gifford, L., 1998. Pain, the tissues and the nervous system: a conceptual model. *Physiotherapy* 84 (1):27–36.

Kasch, H., Qerama, E., Kongsted, A., et al., 2011. The risk assessment score in acute whiplash injury predicts outcome and reflects biopsychosocial factors. *Spine* 36 (25 Suppl):S263–7.

Krumholz, H. M., Ross, J. S., Presler, A. H., et al., 2007. What have we learnt from Vioxx? *BMJ (Clinical Research Ed.)* 334 (7585):120–3.

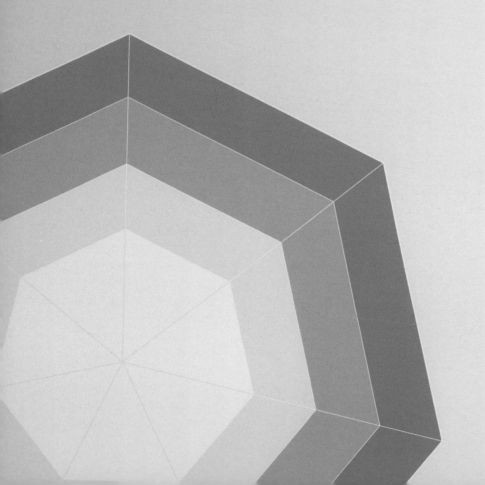

8

The Neuropathic Domain

Overview

A pain experience with a strong neuropathic driver is most easily conceptualized as one in which the tissue that is damaged is neural tissue residing somewhere in the body that is not the brain or spinal cord. Damage to a nerve is often associated with a pain profile that is quite distinct from damage to any other peripheral tissue (e.g. muscle, bone, ligament or tendon). Assuming that you've already cleared the viscera as a potential pain driver in the initial screening, and for the purposes of this section, the remaining peripheral tissues can best be classed as either neural or non-neural, or contractile vs. non-contractile depending on your perspective and intentions.

Neuropathic pain, often abbreviated to *NeP*, is necessarily initiated by damage to a peripheral nerve that affects the manner in which that nerve transmits action potentials across the nerve membrane. The damage will also very likely disrupt the normal flow of intraneural nutrients from terminal to terminal through the intracellular flow of axoplasm (the fluid internal medium of a nerve cell). Damage can be the result of physical trauma (excessive compression, laceration or traction/stretching), a disease process (infection or inflammation) or a change in nutrition or environment around the nerve (e.g. atrophy and degeneration as can occur in unmanaged diabetes). Not considered here, though sharing similarities in clinical presentation, are central nervous system afflictions including central post-stroke (thalamic) pain syndrome, phantom limb pain, and possibly complex regional pain syndrome (CRPS, though we note that the jury is still somewhat out on the balance of peripheral vs. central contributions in CRPS).

There are now defined criteria for identifying neuropathic pain described in the 'Distinguishing features' section below, though consistent to all is that the history of the condition needs to be clearly associated and consistent with peripheral nerve damage or disease. It is worth noting however that as work continues in the field of peripheral and central pain conditions, the distinguishing line between the two is often blurred and it is rare that peripheral neuropathy exists without an associated central mechanism, as described in Chapter 9.

The ability to record activity directly from nerve cells *in vivo* using advanced neurophysiological techniques combined with cellular microscopy for visualization of individual cells has shed increasing light on what happens when an axon is damaged. To fully understand this field requires an appreciation of the anatomy of a nerve for which at least a cursory overview is warranted.

Nerve anatomy

Starting externally, what we commonly think of as a 'nerve' is in fact a collection of fascicles (nerve cells) all wrapped together with blood vessels in a connective membrane called the *epineurium*. The epineurium is an important part of this story as it is non-conductive (non-neural) but instead is itself innervated by smaller nerves called *nervi nervorum* and receives blood supply from a network of thin capillaries called *vasi nervorum*. This is important in that the outer membrane, the epineurium, of a nerve can be damaged (most commonly compressed or stretched) and become inflamed and hyperalgesic (painful) without damage to the actual nerve cells within the sheath. This is NOT neuropathic pain, rather it is better conceptualized as pain that is primarily nociceptive, which is rare and very difficult to identify clinically. A clinical condition called 'entrapment syndrome' may present this way, where the epineurium is adhered to or compressed by surrounding connective tissue leading to traction or compression and inflammation (and pain). The distinguishing features between this kind of entrapment syndrome and neuropathic pain are pain with predictable and consistent movement of the local joints or contraction of the muscles surrounding the joints in entrapment syndrome. However, the criteria for neuropathic pain is not met unless the severity of the entrapment or compression results in damaged axons.

Deep to the epineurium, wrapping a collection of nerve cells into individual *fascicles* is the *perineurium*. Each individual nerve cell itself is wrapped in endoneurium, which effectively delineates each axon from another to prevent cross-talk. This is analogous to household electrical wiring, where an outer sheath protects two or more copper wires within, that themselves are individually wrapped to prevent an electrical short circuit (Fig. 8.1).

Having gone through those connective tissue layers we reach the individual nerve cells that transmit electrical action potentials along their highly excitable nerve membranes. We're making an assumption that most readers will be familiar with at least the general components of a nerve cell, that includes a dendrite (most commonly the part of the cell that contains the primary machinery of cell life such as the nucleus, mitochondria, and other cell components) that may receive input in the form of synaptic neurotransmitters from several neighboring nerves, and an axon that can range in length from very short (a millimeter or less) to very long (the sciatic nerve, if you include its branches, will run a good meter in adult humans). The axon itself is a tube formed by the cell membrane that contains an intracellular milieu of sugars, proteins, ions, and other cell components all flowing within a fluid medium termed axoplasm. The *membrane* is a lipid barrier that separates the internal cell environment from the external cell environment, and is riddled with holes that can open and close, commonly called *gates*. When the cell membrane is at rest, the gates are mostly closed, and the relative concentrations of charged ions, mostly sodium, potassium, and calcium, between the internal and external environments set up a potential difference in charge that, again like household wiring, can be measured in terms of voltage. This is called the 'resting membrane potential', and in most human nerve cells ranges somewhere between -40 and -90 millivolts.

Things get slightly more complex from here, probably beyond where we need to go for our purposes in a book about clinical pain syndromes. To keep it somewhat simple, some of the gates in a nerve membrane will open in response to specific stimuli. These could be chemical, thermal, or mechanical, or some combination of those. These types of gates are usually found at the end (terminals) of an axon, usually called end organs, where they are embedded in the target tissue to allow the nerve to sample (sense) its environment. This being a book about pain, we're going to focus this discussion on *sensory* ('afferent') nerves rather than *motor* (efferent) nerves, though the general processes are fairly similar. As we described in Chapter 7 on nociceptive drivers, if a sensory nerve is exposed to the 'right' stimulus at the 'right' intensity, then those specialized channels will open. When the channels open, the ion imbalance rapidly tries to correct itself, usually with an exchange of sodium and potassium ions between the intra- and extracellular media, to reach a state of electrical equilibrium termed 'depolarization'. The entire axonal membrane is full of gated channels that are sensitive to local changes in voltage, so when one gate opens and depolarizes its part of the membrane, neighboring gates will sense that and open to depolarize *their* part of the membrane. Nature being what it is, there are plenty of redundant gates within the cell membrane that aren't needed for passing the action along the nerve membrane so they are usually covered by another, non-excitable membrane called the *myelin sheath*. The sheath covers most gates, exposing only enough to ensure that action potentials can be reliably and rapidly propagated along the membrane. Since the action potential skips several gates, it is said to 'jump' along the membrane in a process called *saltatory conduction* (from the Latin *saltare*, to hop or leap; Fig. 8.2). This process of consecutively depolarizing areas of membrane skips along the nerve cell until it terminates usually at the spinal cord. From there the action is handed over to the spinal cord neuron, and the process carries on up to the brain for interpretation, perception, and awareness.

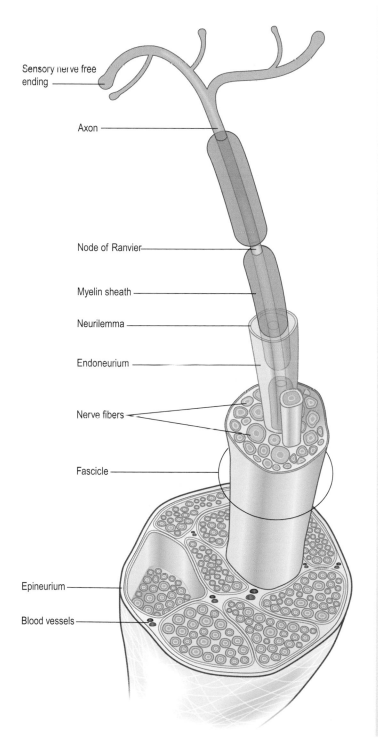

Sensory nerve free ending

Axon

Node of Ranvier

Myelin sheath

Neurilemma

Endoneurium

Nerve fibers

Fascicle

Epineurium

Blood vessels

Figure 8.1
A cross-section of a peripheral nerve showing the different layers of neural and connective tissues. Starting from the individual sensory afferent or motor efferent, we see the myelin sheath (Schwann cells) wrapped in endoneurium, then grouped together with other similar afferents or efferents in perineurium as a fascicle, with several fascicles wrapped in epineurium as a full nerve.

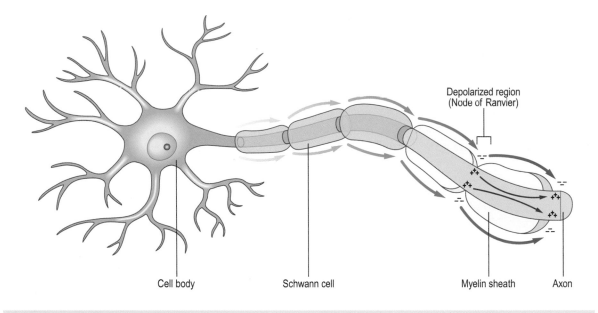

Depolarized region
(Node of Ranvier)

Cell body   Schwann cell   Myelin sheath   Axon

Figure 8.2
A diagrammatic representation of saltatory conduction. Schwann cells create a sheath of lipid myelin that have gaps at regular intervals. Membrane depolarization occurs at the gaps meaning action potentials travel much faster from axon to dendrite or dendrite to axon.

Proposed mechanisms

That was a somewhat superficial overview of how action potentials propagate along a nerve cell membrane but was necessary background for making sense of neuropathic pain. While there is probably no single mechanism for explaining the peculiar and unpleasant symptoms of neuropathic pain, research has uncovered several potential mechanisms. When a nerve is completely cut or transected (sometimes called 'neurotmesis'), all of the axons within and all of the connective tissue around them, have been completely cut off from the rest of the nerve distal to the transection. This means all sorts of things, not least of which is that the brain, whose only connection to the rest of the body is through the nerves, loses all ability to receive information from, or send information to, the area innervated by the cut nerve. If this is a mixed

nerve (containing both motor and sensory fibers), then the intuitive result would be numbness in the area (sensory information can't get in) and paralysis of the innervated muscles (motor drive can't get out). On its own that would be bad enough but remembering that the nerve membrane serves a very important function of keeping the internal and external environments separate, a completely cut nerve means that all ability to manage the flow of action potentials is gone. To use our electrical wiring analogy, the nerve is now sparking like an out-of-control live wire, at least until the 'bare' cut end can be closed again and resting membrane potential re-established. The impulses flow rapidly back to the central nervous system, not because of something happening in the target tissue but because of the now uninhibited nerve that would normally be innervating it. Of course, all the brain receives is electrical impulses, it gets no information about *where* on the nerve that information is originating. As a result the interpretation of the information will be that something terrible is happening to, say, the left 1½ fingers, but in reality that's only the area to which the brain is assigning the problem because all it perceives is a sudden flurry of information coming in from the 'left 1½ fingers nerve' (left ulnar nerve in this example).

That is a somewhat extreme example of what happens with nerve damage, but complete transection is not necessary for neuropathy. Any process that leads to degeneration of the myelin sheath will usually be enough to cause some kind of strange sensation, ranging from numbness and tingling, to pins and needles, to chills, electrical 'shocks', or unrelenting burning pain in the unfortunate few. Whether due to action potentials that don't 'flow' properly along the nerve membrane (lost saltatory conduction), membrane gates that are now exposed and active when they shouldn't be (leading to mid-nerve depolarization called 'ectopic' potentials), or constriction of the axoplasmic flow that delivers nutrients and transmitters to the distal parts of the nerve, the information being received from the brain is no longer an accurate representation of what's happening in the tissues. As the pressure, infection, or traction carries on, immune and inflammatory processes kick in that can *really* make things weird. Neighboring axons or full nerves may be exposed to new inflammatory messengers and themselves become inflamed or active, leading to an experience of pain potentially spreading across normal boundaries of nerve innervation. Further, as axons lose their nutrition they begin to degenerate through a process called Wallerian degeneration, leaving openings in nerve terminals that may at least temporarily be 'plugged' by neighboring nerves. Sometimes bare axons where myelin has been degraded will sprout new limbs to connect with

neighboring axons. If they're all high-threshold sensory nerves, then the result is most likely to be that the patient experiences non-dermatomal spreading pain. There is some controversy about whether this now still classifies as 'neuropathic pain', as the current diagnostic guidelines require that the symptoms be felt along the known anatomical distribution of a nerve, but we'll leave readers to use their own judgment in making this call.

If we follow this logic, it is possible to understand the many hypotheses that have been presented to explain the often strange symptoms associated with neuropathy. As recently as a decade ago, one popular hypothesis was that low-threshold 'touch-sensitive' sensory nerves (e.g. Aβ fibers) may sprout axonal limbs to either connect directly to a neighboring damaged high-threshold nociceptive nerve (e.g. C fibers) or to the spinal cord laminae most often reserved for nociceptive input. The hypothesis went that this sort of cross-talk between low-threshold and high-threshold nerves meant that light touch could be interpreted by the brain as pain. This phenomenon is termed *allodynia* and is a common feature of neuropathic pain, though more recent evidence using advanced staining and analysis techniques has not supported this hypothesis (e.g. Zhang et al., 2015). Another hypothesis that has more support is that rather than cross-talk between nerves of different thresholds, the damaged nerve undergoes an observable phenotypic transformation through which, say, a previously high-threshold nociceptive afferent now functions more like a low-threshold touch afferent (i.e. responds to different stimuli, releases different neurotransmitters) (Berger et al., 2011). In this hypothesis, the pre-trauma connections remain unchanged, but the behavior of the peripheral nerve has changed. Ectopic discharge, loss of inhibitory control, and neuroinflammation are other hypotheses that continue to be explored to better understand the mechanisms of, and identify treatment targets for, neuropathic pain.

Regardless of the mechanism, neuropathic pain is probably most easily conceptualized as a condition of *disinhibition*, in that the peripheral nervous system has lost the ability to effectively control or modulate input to the spinal cord and brain. However, there are many examples of an 'inhibitory' presentation (or perhaps, 'de-facilitated', just to make it even more complicated) where the primary signs and symptoms are coolness of the skin, muscle atrophy, and full or partial paralysis. This story will become clearer as research advances, and we will revisit some of these differences when we get to the central nociplastic drivers of pain in Chapter 9.

Distinguishing features

There have been (very) many sets of diagnostic criteria published for identifying neuropathic pain over the years, but we're going to focus on those of Finnerup and colleagues from 2016 (Finnerup et al., 2016; Fig. 8.3) as they have also largely been adopted by the International Association for the Study of Pain (IASP). They also overlap quite closely with the criteria set forth by van Hecke and colleagues (van Hecke et al., 2015), which were arguably more rigorously developed but also targeted more for use in identifying cases and controls for genetic research.

The first pass for screening in this protocol is in two parts: **Step 1** is that the presentation *has to have been preceded by a lesion or disease process* that could have logically led to damage of a nerve or, since the authors include central post-stroke pain and trigeminal neuralgia, a central nerve system. **Step 2** is that the pain *must be present* in a region that is "neuroanatomically plausible", plausibility in this case referring to pain where you'd think it would be felt given the type of disease or lesion. This is somewhat ambiguous,

though see Table 8.1 for a list of common anatomical sites that would be expected in most neuropathic pain syndromes.

If the mechanisms and distribution of pain seem logical, then neuropathic pain is 'possible'.

The second pass on this protocol is that there are other associated signs or symptoms that are in or around that same 'neurologically plausible' distribution. Here one can get slightly creative, as neuropathic pain has been associated with a whole host of signs and symptoms. These could include symptoms described as burning, freezing, shock-like, heavy, numb, itching, crawling, or others. Sensory loss (paresthesia) is usually required, though the presence of touch- or thermally-evoked allodynia also counts. Cold hyperalgesia (increased sensitivity to cold stimuli) is a commonly recognized clinical sign in neuropathic pain that can be tested either using simple tools like a test tube filled with ice water, an ice cube in a plastic bag, or a cold metal rod. Lab-based measurement tools are also available, such as the TSA-II Neurosensory Analyzer from Medoc Inc. (Israel) (Fig. 8.4), though these are not cost-efficient for most clinical practices. Both the Finnerup and the van Hecke groups suggest using a standardized self-report screening tool here, of which a few have been designed (see table below). If you find weird and wacky symptoms on top of the two steps from stage 1, then this is "probable" neuropathic pain. For a "definite" neuropathic pain call, you need the highest level of evidence which requires objective findings from diagnostic testing. Depending on the nature of the condition, this could include imaging, skin biopsy, microneurography, or surgical verification of a lesion. As we're focusing this book on the non-specialist clinical environment, these diagnostic techniques will not be further explored.

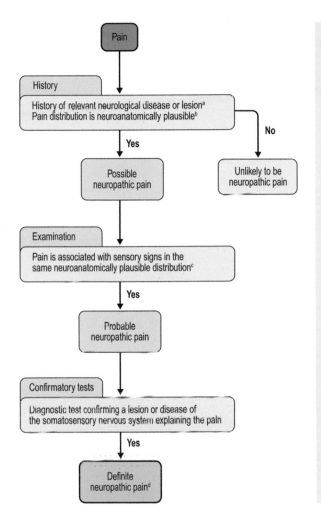

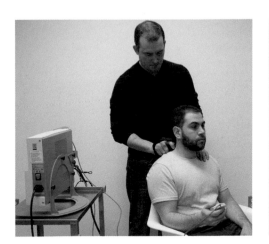

Figure 8.3
Flow chart of updated grading system for neuropathic pain.
[a]History, including pain descriptors, the presence of nonpainful sensory symptoms, and aggravating and alleviating factors, suggestive of pain being related to a neurological lesion and not other causes such as inflammation or non-neural tissue damage. The suspected lesion or disease is reported to be associated with neuropathic pain, including a temporal and spatial relationship representative of the condition; includes paroxysmal pain in trigeminal neuralgia.
[b]The pain distribution reported by the patient is consistent with the suspected lesion or disease (Table 8.1).
[c]The area of sensory changes may extend beyond, be within, or overlap with the area of pain. Sensory loss is generally required but touch-evoked or thermal allodynia may be the only finding at bedside examination. Trigger phenomena in trigeminal neuralgia may be counted as sensory signs. In some cases, sensory signs may be difficult to demonstrate although the nature of the lesion or disease is confirmed; for these cases the level "probable" continues to be appropriate, if a diagnostic test confirms the lesion or disease of the somatosensory nervous system.
[d]The term "definite" in this context means "probable neuropathic pain with confirmatory tests" because the location and nature of the lesion or disease have been confirmed to be able to explain the pain. "Definite" neuropathic pain is a pain that is fully compatible with neuropathic pain, but it does not necessarily establish causality.
(Reproduced with permission from Finnerup, N.B., Haroutounian, S., Kamerman, P., et al., 2016. Neuropathic pain: an updated grading system for research and clinical practice. *Pain* 157(8):1599–606.)

Figure 8.4
Example of a method for testing thermal sensitivity/thermal pain threshold. The TSA-II Neurosensory Analyzer (Medoc, Inc.) can be used for this purpose. A thermode is applied to the skin over the area to be tested. The thermode can be either heated or cooled at 1°C per second. The patient is asked to push the button at the moment the sensation becomes painful. This is a pricey option for a tool that may be used infrequently. We have had some success using a simpler test: a large construction nail with the pointed end wrapped in tape and stored in a standard residential freezer. Application of the cold metal to the skin can be rated on an intensity scale of 0–10 or 0–20 (where 0 = no sensation, 10 or 20 = extremely painful). We've found that those who rate 13/20 (7/10) or higher can be considered to have cold hyperalgesia, though this has yet to be rigorously explored through research.

Table 8.1 Common neuropathic pain conditions and neuroanatomically plausible distribution of pain symptoms and sensory signs

Neuropathic pain condition	Neuroanatomically plausible distribution of pain and sensory signs	Illustration of typical distribution
Trigeminal neuralgia	Within the facial or intraoral trigeminal territory.	
Postherpetic neuralgia	Unilateral distributed in one or more spinal dermatomes or the trigeminal ophthalmic division.	
Peripheral nerve injury pain	In the innervation territory of the lesioned nerve, typically distal to a trauma, surgery, or compression.	
Postamputation pain	In the missing body part and/or in the residual limb.	
Painful polyneuropathy	In the feet, may extend to involve lower legs, thighs and hands.	

Table 8.1 Common neuropathic pain conditions and neuroanatomically plausible distribution of pain symptoms and sensory signs *continued*

Neuropathic pain condition	Neuroanatomically plausible distribution of pain and sensory signs	Illustration of typical distribution
Painful radiculopathy	Distribution consistent with the innervation territory of the nerve root.	
Neuropathic pain associated with spinal cord injury	At and/or below the level of the spinal cord lesion.	
Central poststroke pain	Contralateral to the stroke. In lateral medullary infarction, the distribution can also involve the ipsilatreral side of the face.	
Central neuropathic pain associated with multiple sclerosis	Can be a combination of distributions seen in spinal cord injury and stroke.	

Reproduced with permission from Finnerup, N.B., Haroutounian, S., Kamerman, P., et al., 2016. Neuropathic pain: an updated grading system for research and clinical practice. *Pain* 157(8):1599–606.

Chapter 8

Suggested evidence for triangulation: neuropathic domain		
Test domains	**Findings**	**Shift in likelihood**
Screening tools	Several have been designed, though the most recognizable are: the Self-report version of the Leeds Assessment of Neuropathic Signs and Symptoms (S-LANSS), the Douleur Neuropathique-4 (DN4), the ID Pain, the PainDETECT, and the Neuropathic Pain Questionnaire. A 2015 review by Mathieson and colleagues (Mathieson et al., 2015) found that almost all are more specific than sensitive, meaning a high score is useful for screening NeP but a low score may be a false negative.	If score is 'high' (as defined by the existing literature): ++
Symptom behavior	Inconsistent, usually without an obvious mechanical pattern, but should be present, ideally confined, to a region of innervation by a potentially damaged peripheral nerve. Could be pain at rest as easily as pain with movement. Symptoms descriptors are also often 'paroxysmal', including shooting, tingling, itching, or shock-like. While this may be useful for discriminating from nociceptive drivers, there will be some overlap here with more central drivers.	++
Palpation	Hyperalgesia (sensitivity to palpation) is common as per many pain conditions, though the presence of identifiable 'tender' or 'trigger' points in muscle is less likely than in a nociceptive driver. A key distinguishing feature is a report of pain in response to a normally non-noxious stimulus, like light pressure (static) or light brushing (dynamic). This phenomenon, termed allodynia, may also be present with a central pain driver, but when present in a region innervated by a damaged nerve it is a hallmark of neuropathic pain.	+ (++ if allodynia present)
Quantitative sensory testing	Expect abnormalities in almost all sensory stimuli, though pressure (mechanical) pain detection threshold may be the least discriminative here. Thermal hyperalgesia (cold or heat, see Fig. 8.4) is common, as would be loss of fine touch (Fig. 8.5), vibratory or electrical (current) detection sensitivity especially in inhibited/de-facilitated neuropathy. There is evidence that 'wind-up' pain, intended as an indicator of abnormal temporal summation of action potentials, is also diagnostic for NeP but also appears to be common with more of a central driver. Once again, the sensory abnormalities must be present within the region of skin innervated by a peripheral nerve or nerves likely to have been injured to be considered neuropathic.	+ if only mechanical hyperalgesia, ++ if thermal hyperalgesia
Sensorimotor testing	The nature of sensorimotor findings will be influenced by the nature and extent of the damaged peripheral nerves. Proprioceptive deficits are unlikely here, though conditions with involvement of motor nerves should be expected to show signs of weakness or partial paralysis of the muscles innervated by the damaged nerve. Other paroxysmal symptoms such as a feeling of 'fullness' in the area innervated by the damaged nerve or feeling that the area is swollen when it visibly (and objectively) is not could be part of the experience of NeP but also overlaps with central or sensorimotor drivers.	+

Suggested evidence for triangulation: neuropathic domain *continued*

Test domains	Findings	Shift in likelihood
Mechanical testing	Consistent mechanical signs are unlikely here, though tests that apply tension to known peripheral nerves may be positive (e.g. upper limb neurodynamic tests, lower limb tests such as the passive or crossed straight leg raise). As these are also potentially positive in cases of nerve tethering or adhesions without damage (non-neuropathic), they should be considered supportive evidence for triangulation rather than discriminative on their own.	+
Cognitions	Considerable evidence indicates that those with neuropathic pain problems will also provide more negative responses on questionnaires of pain-related cognitions. However, that is not to say that these cognitions are drivers of neuropathic pain, rather the experience of living with neuropathic pain, that is often constant, unpredictable, and severe, would quite rationally lead one to worry about their symptoms and have difficulty thinking about things other than the pain. So, while it should be expected that people with a neuropathic driver score high on tools of pain-related cognitions, this should not be inherently taken to indicate irrational beliefs or that those beliefs are themselves the pain driver.	Neutral
Emotions	Similar to cognitions, there is a large body of evidence to indicate that people with neuropathic pain also tend to rate quality of life lower than average and score higher on tools that screen for things like depression and anxiety. It is certainly possible that psychopathology is contributing to the experience of neuropathic pain, but emotional screens should not be considered diagnostic for this driver.	Neutral
Socioenviron-mental	There is very little evidence to indicate how, if at all, socioenvironmental aspects contribute to, or can be used to screen for, NeP. The Global Burden of Disease studies do not specifically track NeP so it is difficult to state with confidence if it's more prevalent in certain countries or cultures than others. However, some mechanisms of NeP, such as cancer (with/without chemotherapy), diabetes, HIV, herpes (varicella) zoster infection, sickle cell anemia, malnutrition or others, most likely have regional and cultural differences that may contribute to identifying a likely neuropathic driver. A simple example would be post-herpetic neuralgia, the risk for which increases with age. Socioeconomic status, access to good food and clean water, exercise and activity habits, socioeconomic status and cultural influences on healthcare-seeking, including attitudes and access, all likely have a role to play as moderators of the likelihood of a neuropathic pain driver, but are not in themselves diagnostic or discriminative.	Neutral
Pathology	An important part of the identification of a neuropathic driver is the etiology. For a diagnosis of NeP in most guidelines, the onset of symptoms needs to be associated with physical damage (crush, traction, or laceration), infection, inflammation, or disease likely affecting a peripheral nerve. Verification through imaging, biopsy, or electrodiagnosis can be useful here, but the history of damage is required.	++

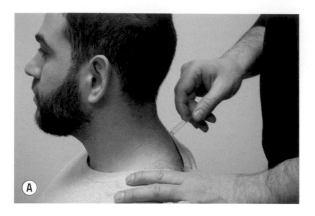
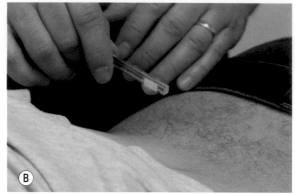

Figure 8.5
Example of testing fine touch over the skin of the neck (**A**) and low back (**B**). A monofilament is touched to the skin with enough pressure to make it bend. The patient is asked to indicate when they feel the filament. Monofilaments come in different 'weights' (stiffness) and normative data are available for testing at several different body sites for comparison against normal sensation.

Prognostic value

The prognosis of pain with a primarily neuropathic driver, or any pain with neuropathy-like symptoms, is generally not good. Our own work and that of our colleagues has shown that people with post-traumatic neck pain (whiplash) who score high on the S-LANSS tool are more likely to rate themselves as not recovered three to six months later and are less likely to respond to rehabilitation interventions. The same appears to be true for low back pain that has *neuropathy-like symptoms*. Some mechanisms of neuropathic pain, such as acute herpes zoster infection (shingles) may do well with antiviral therapies if caught early, though even then there are around 2% of people who will develop long-term painful post-herpetic neuralgia. Most estimates of recovery from conditions such as axonotmesis (axonal transection with surrounding sheath still intact) have been driven by clinical anecdote and experience rather than empiricism, with a common explanation that nerves 'heal' (regenerate) at a rate of about 1 cm per month. It's hard to find evidence to support that explanation, and it is most likely used as a simple frame of reference for discussing expectations with patients rather than anything grounded in basic or clinical science. Even then, a fully healed nerve is not an automatic ticket out of neuropathic pain, whose symptoms may persist after objective signs of healing. Complete transection (neurotmesis) of a peripheral nerve may never heal, and in some cases could lead to an experience of pain better conceptualized as a sort of quasi-phantom limb pain, blurring the lines between peripheral neuropathy and more central mechanisms.

In empirical terms, a 2015 systematic review by Boogaard and colleagues (Boogaard et al., 2015) found that most of the evidence came from post-herpetic neuralgia (PHN), with few high quality studies at the time to help clinicians identify those unlikely to recover from peripheral neuropathy (sciatica), post-surgical pain, or other types of neuropathy. For PHN, predictors of persistent problems (non-recovery) included male sex, older age, smoking history, higher severity of symptoms like pain or rash, not taking antiviral medications, and overall poor general health status. From a single high-quality study on sciatica/ peripheral neuropathy, they found that cognitive factors such as negative expectations for recovery, fear of movement, and a preference for passive coping strategies were predictive of non-recovery. It seems that more research would be beneficial here to help clinicians better understand both the influence of neuropathic signs and symptoms on recovery from pain, and the effect of other patient characteristics on recovery from neuropathy.

Intervention strategies

Intervention for neuropathic pain is most commonly initiated pharmaceutically, with gabapentin or pregabalin currently considered first-line therapies, with or without an opioid. Physical and/or psychological therapies are also often prescribed where available. Physical therapies may include advice around modifying daily activities to optimize function, education about the nature of pain and neuropathy, and light active movements usually without resistance (though some have found benefit from resisted movements in water). Desensitization protocols, especially where sensory hypersensitivity is present, have been met with mixed results, and physical agents such as transcutaneous electrical nerve stimulation or acupuncture have similarly mixed or small effects. Most clinicians will attempt to avoid movements or activities that tension the injured nerve, though there are times where 'nerve flossing' techniques may be of value especially in more chronic neuropathy where nerve tethering is suspected. Psychological interventions tend to focus on cognitive reframing of painful sensations, effective coping strategies, cognitive behavioral techniques, or acceptance and commitment therapies where full recovery is unexpected but some function can still

be performed. Occasionally, psychological or psychiatric intervention for emotional interference like depression is required, and there is some evidence that common antidepressant medications like tricyclic antidepressants (TCAs), selective serotonin reuptake inhibitors (SSRIs) or serotonin noradrenaline reuptake inhibitors (SNRIs) may provide some relief of neuropathic pain symptoms in the right patients (Lee & Chen, 2010). In most cases a multimodal interprofessional approach is the preferred model for helping patients manage neuropathic pain.

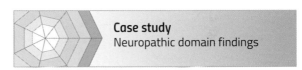

Case study
Neuropathic domain findings

Returning to our case of Sean, there is already enough information from what we've collected so far to triangulate the peripheral neuropathic domain as a very low relative driver of his pain experience. While the mechanism of injury (traumatic neck injury) *could* be consistent with the possibility of some cervical nerve compression or brachial plexus traction, there are no additional signs or symptoms that point to this domain. His clinical neurological exam for peripheral nerve function (lower motor neuron, sensory) is largely normal, he does not describe neuropathic-type symptoms like tingling, electric-like, itching, cold or others, and there is no indication that his symptoms are restricted to the known distribution of a peripheral nerve. While the occasional radiating symptoms into the upper arm may be a small piece of evidence, this would also fit with known patterns of referred pain from cervical or shoulder girdle injury.

So, while it is not necessary to collect further information for this domain (saving us time and reducing burden to Sean), for the sake of this case example, let's say we had Sean complete the Self-report version of the Leeds Assessment for Neuropathic Signs and Symptoms (S-LANSS) and he scored a 4/24, well below the threshold of 12/24 for identifying pain of primarily neuropathic origin (POPNO). By this time additional testing is clearly not necessary, and we'll leave that point on the radar plot at 'low to very low' (Fig. 8.6).

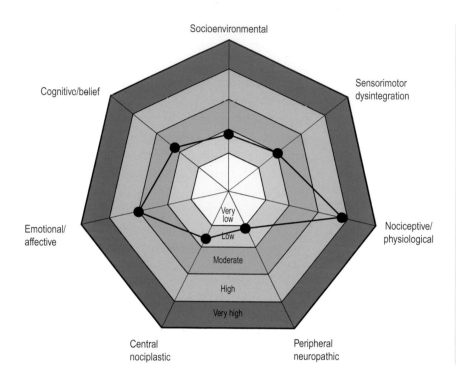

Figure 8.6
Sean's radar plot continues to take shape. Based on the neuropathic domain findings, this driver has been kept at 'very low' probability.

References

Berger, J. V., Knaepen, L., Janssen, S. P., et al., 2011. Cellular and molecular insights into neuropathy-induced pain hypersensitivity for mechanism-based treatment approaches. *Brain Research Reviews* 67 (1–2):282–310.

Boogaard, S., Heymans, M. W., de Vet, H. C., et al., 2015. Predictors of persistent neuropathic pain –a systematic review. *Pain physician* 18 (5):433–57.

Finnerup, N. B., Haroutounian, S., Kamerman, P., et al., 2016. Neuropathic pain: an updated grading system for research and clinical practice. *Pain* 157 (8):1599–606.

Lee, Y.-C., Chen, P.-P., 2010. A review of SSRIs and SNRIs in neuropathic pain. *Expert Opinion on Pharmacotherapy* 11 (17):2813–25.

Mathieson, S., Maher, C. G., Terwee, C. B., et al., 2015. Neuropathic pain screening questionnaires have limited measurement properties. A systematic review. *Journal of Clinical Epidemiology* 68 (8):957–66.

van Hecke, O., Kamerman, P. R., Attal, N., et al., 2015. Neuropathic pain phenotyping by international consensus (NeuroPPIC) for genetic studies: a NeuPSIG systematic review, Delphi survey, and expert panel recommendations. *Pain* 156 (11):2337–53.

Zhang, Y., Chen, Y., Liedtke, W., et al., 2015. Lack of evidence for ectopic sprouting of genetically labeled Aβ touch afferents in inflammatory and neuropathic trigeminal pain. *Molecular Pain* 11:18.

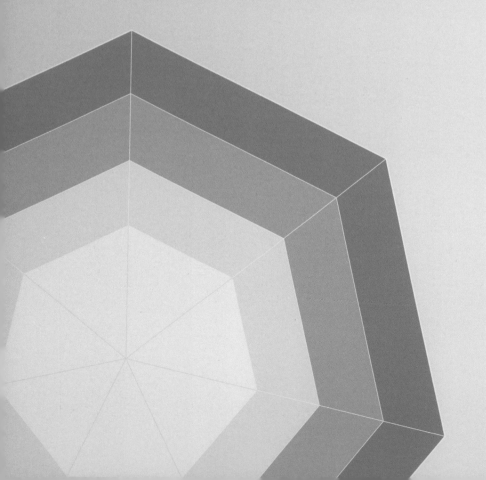

9

The Central Nociplastic Domain

Proposed mechanisms

This domain currently represents arguably one of the most active fields of research in pain science. The ubiquitous term *central sensitization* has given rise to several new ways of thinking about the phenomenon of centrally maintained or centrally generated pain, with terms such as facilitation, disinhibition, descending inhibitory control, neuroplasticity, phenotypic plasticity, algopathy, and nociplastic change, among others, appearing in the literature. While we will stop short of endorsing one term over another, we feel it would be helpful to use and stick with one term. We have chosen *nociplastic,* a term coined by a group led by Prof. Kathleen Sluka at the University of Iowa, serving as an umbrella term for changes in the function or structure of the central nervous system (CNS, comprised of the spinal cord and brain) that can maintain pain in the absence of peripheral tissue damage. The term fits our understanding of the phenomenon, though it is not yet universally accepted. Whether *nociplastic* sticks and becomes widely acknowledged remains to be seen, but IASP has officially endorsed it so we expect it will eventually become part of the standard lexicon. We encourage you to keep an eye on these developments.

So, let's embrace the challenge of pulling all of the emerging knowledge from such an active field together in a practical and consistent manner for the purpose of understanding a central nociplastic driver of a patient's pain experience. The simplest way to conceptualize the concept of a nociplastic driver is as a pain experience that is no longer driven by ongoing processes (damage, inflammation) from the periphery but rather is driven or maintained by activity occurring in the CNS. There are almost as many hypotheses as there are researchers in the field investigating how this process comes to pass, and we cannot, nor do we intend to, do justice to them all. There are some consistencies however that we can draw upon. In most that do not include a disease process (e.g. stroke or CNS infection), the etiology is often thought to at least be initiated by some kind of input from the periphery, though even that is contentious and not consistently accepted. What is generally accepted with some degree of agreement is that the activation properties of neurons of the spinal cord or brain can be modified either through persistent (tonic) input from peripheral nerves, or through immune or inflammatory activity in the CNS itself, such as occurs when glial cells (astrocytes, oligodendrocytes, or microglia) are activated (Box 9.1).

The nature of these nociplastic modifications appear to vary widely. In some cases, it looks as if neurons normally involved in transmitting nociceptive information become responsive to, and express membrane receptors for, neurotransmitters normally reserved for light touch or thermal information, such that they are activated when impulses from non-noxious stimuli reach the spinal cord. Other research evidence indicates that the spinal cord neurons normally responsible for transmitting high-threshold nociceptive information reduce their activation thresholds (go from high-threshold to medium- or low-threshold) such that less intense information (e.g. less frequent impulses or less input from multiple peripheral nerves) results in a depolarization of their membranes sending action potentials on up to the brain.

The central nervous system is also full of inhibitory interneurons, meaning that it might be more appropriate to consider the central nervous system as always active but with inhibitory barriers in place that prevent unwanted activity (rather than a dormant blob waiting to be activated). In this view, centrally maintained pain may be the result of inhibitory

---

Box 9.1 Factors that could activate glial cells

- Peripheral nerve injury (compression, traction, chemical)
- Physical trauma
- Psychological trauma or distress
- Hypoxia/ischemia
- Infections
- Toxins

checkpoints that become less effective, meaning more information gets through to the brain where, under normal circumstances, it would have not reached threshold for propagation. Those glial cells we mentioned above may also play a role here. Researchers have shown that when peripheral tissues are damaged, inflammatory mediators can enter the nerve axoplasm and be transported towards the CNS. There they are released from the dendritic spines, and the normally dormant glial cells can be activated in response to these *proinflammatory cytokines*. When activated, the immune functions of glial cells kick in and they themselves begin to release those same (or similar) proinflammatory cytokines. In a somewhat self-perpetuating cycle, the glial cells then sensitize the very nerves that activated them in the first place (Fig. 9.1). Even when information stops coming in from the periphery, it appears that under some circumstances glial activation can maintain the firing of the spinal cord neurons.

The brain is also subject to change from nociceptive input, and there is now a large accumulation of evidence in the field to show that, for example, the brains of some people with chronic pain look different, both structurally and functionally, than the brains of their healthy matched controls. Much of this work started in the late 1990s with the advent and accessibility of positron emission tomography (PET) scanning of the brain. One of the earlier pioneers, Dr. Herta Flor who remains active in the field as of this writing, used PET scans to show that stimulation of the skin of the low back in people with chronic low back pain led to activity in the somatosensory cortex of the brain, not only the region generally associated with the back, but also in the region more associated with representations of the leg (Flor et al., 1997). The same activation pattern was not present in healthy matched controls, showing for one of the first times that the experience of living

with chronic low back pain may in fact change the processing of sensory stimuli from the periphery. It also provided a rather interesting alternative explanation for the experience of radiating leg pain in those with chronic back pain – until then, it had been assumed that radiating leg pain was a result of sciatic nerve compression, but this evidence in the brain could suggest that leg pain is a function of brain plasticity rather than anything to do with the sciatic nerve.

PET scanning is a somewhat burdensome process and requires the injection of a radioactive dye, so it was not widely used in pain research. Shortly following Dr. Flor's initial work however, a new imaging technology called functional magnetic resonance imaging (fMRI) emerged and completely changed the way scientists were able to 'see' activity in the brain without injecting anything into patients or exposing them to ionizing radiation, which would be the case with PET. fMRI is a tremendous achievement of modern engineering, using the known magnetic properties of water molecules to image the amount of activity occurring in the brain of a person inside the MRI machine in real time.[1] This technology has led to tremendous advancements within and certainly beyond pain research, to the point that some would even say we can estimate the amount of pain someone is actually experiencing based on the activity in their brain on fMRI. That is a topic fraught with contention, differing views, and considerable medical, ethical, and legal implications, much of which were summarized nicely by a team of leaders in the field in a 2017 article in the top journal *Nature* including Dr. Flor herself (Davis et al., 2017).

While the topic of whether it is possible to objectively and accurately quantify pain through brain imaging is highly contentious, more widely accepted is that fMRI when used properly has revealed that

---

[1] In actuality that's not entirely accurate; fMRI captures the flow of blood in and out of different brain regions (termed 'regional cerebral blood flow'), with the understanding that those regions of the brain that are using more blood are more neurologically active.

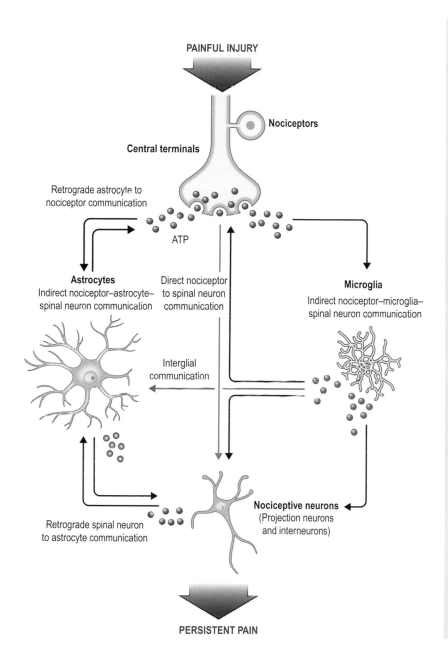

PAINFUL INJURY

Nociceptors

Central terminals

Retrograde astrocyte to
nociceptor communication

ATP

Astrocytes
Indirect nociceptor–astrocyte–
spinal neuron communication

Direct nociceptor
to spinal neuron
communication

Microglia
Indirect nociceptor–microglia–
spinal neuron communication

Interglial
communication

Retrograde spinal neuron
to astrocyte communication

Nociceptive neurons
(Projection neurons
and interneurons)

PERSISTENT PAIN

Figure 9.1
Diagrammatic representation of glial activation. Astrocytes and microglia express membrane receptors for some classes of immune and inflammatory mediators and neurotransmitters. When activated, the glial cells generate and release their own chemical mediators that themselves can sensitize or depolarize central neurons. In this model, an amalgam of work from prior authors, *adenosine triphosphate* (ATP) is one of the transmitters released from the terminals of an incoming peripheral nerve. ATP (and others) can directly activate central post-synaptic neurons, but also activate glial cells (astrocytes and microglia). The cascade of events can then lead to the glia themselves releasing their own (ATP-like) transmitters that communicate with one another, with the post-synaptic neuron, or even back to the peripheral nociceptive afferent in a retrograde manner. The latter may be responsible for the phenomenon of 'neurogenic inflammation', where inflammatory mediators are transported back through the nerve cell to the peripheral tissue, and lead to inflammation there.

certain brain regions tend to respond differently to pain stimuli in people with low back pain compared to those without. Common brain regions include those associated with reward and conditioned learning, working and emotional memories, bodily sensory processing, and higher order executive functioning (Fig. 9.2). In some regions of the brain, activity seems to be increased in response to painful stimuli or images, in other areas it is decreased, compared to people without chronic pain.

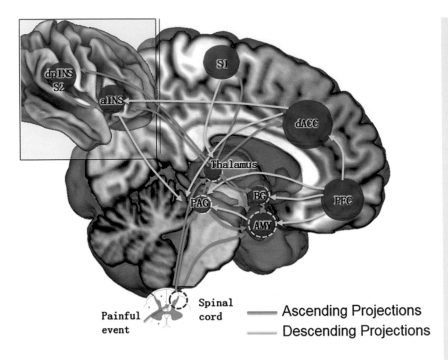

Figure 9.2
The 'Pain Matrix' and its descending modulation. Simplified overview of the brain targets of the ascending (green) and descending (yellow) modulatory pathways for pain. The 'pain matrix' is comprised of the thalamus, anterior cingulate cortex (ACC), the anterior and dorsal posterior insula (aINS and dpINS), primary and secondary somatosensory cortices (S1 and S2) and the periaqueductal gray (PAG), and is often extended to include prefrontal cortices (PFC), as well as the basal ganglia (BG) and amygdala (AMY). Neuroimaging approaches to the study of these pathways must account for the complex interactions between these regions and the multiple roles any one region may play in pain perception. (Reproduced with permission from Reddan, M.C., Wager, T.D. Modeling Pain Using fMRI: From Regions to Biomarkers. *Neuroscience Bulletin* 34(1):208–15. Copyright Shanghai Institutes for Biological Sciences, CAS and Springer Nature Singapore Pte Ltd. 2017.)

Brain structure is another area that has been explored in chronic pain conditions. Evidence accumulated through the first decade of the 2000s showed that the gray matter volume and/or density of people with chronic pain tended to be reduced compared to age-matched controls. In one study (Kuchinad et al., 2007) it was suggested that the thinning of cortical gray matter made the brains of people with fibromyalgia look about 10–20 years older than they actually were. This of course raised interesting questions such as: what are the underlying mechanisms? Are people with congenitally thinner gray matter more vulnerable to chronic pain, or does chronic pain lead to thinner gray matter? Can this be reversed? If yes, how, and would that lead to less pain? Answers to some of these questions started to appear near the end of the 2000s, with one of the first papers coming from Rodriguez-Raecke and colleagues in 2009 who showed that, amongst a group of 10 patients with hip pain, all of whom experienced complete pain relief after a joint replacement, their thinned gray matter started to thicken again (Rodriguez-Raecke et al., 2009).

This was again found in a report published in 2011 by Seminowicz and colleagues who found that in a sample of 14 patients with chronic low back pain, successful surgery was associated with an increase in their previously thinned gray matter six months later (Seminowicz et al., 2011). So, while it seems that living with chronic pain takes a toll on the body and the brain, there are reasons for optimism in that successful intervention may reverse many of those changes. This is another reason we prefer the term nociplastic, as it suggests change is possible.

Melzack and Wall's Gate Control Theory in 1965 suggested that information from the periphery could be very different from that received and interpreted by the brain, leading many leaders in the field to opine that pain is not an accurate representation of what is actually happening in the tissues, and that nociception is neither necessary nor sufficient for pain to be experienced. So, whether it is thinned (and presumably less resourceful) cortical gray matter, regions of the brain that are more or less active than they ought to be, spinal cord neurons that are disinhibited, glial cells that themselves are stimulating action potentials, or any number of potential other mechanisms, the central nociplastic domain is a complex thing to understand and treat. *Some* degree of a centrally sensitized nociceptive system is probably at least a part driver of most (all) chronic pain conditions. It may also play a role in modifying the experience of acute pain. While daunting, as we're about to see, there are also an increasing number of clinical tools to identify and intervene in pain with a strong central nociplastic driver.

Distinguishing features

As both central nociplastic and peripheral neuropathic drivers include a component of nerves not functioning properly, there will be some overlap in signs and symptoms. However, one of the easiest distinctions to make is that pain with a strong central nociplastic driver is not confined to the anatomical region of innervation of a peripheral nerve in the same way neuropathic pain is. Pain with a central nociplastic driver is also not as likely to demonstrate those paroxysmal symptoms associated with neuropathy, including regional numbness and tingling, shock-like, itching pains or crawling sensations, or freezing or burning pains. Because of the facilitated/disinhibited nature of the mechanisms at play, people with pain of a primarily central driver can be expected to demonstrate hyperalgesia (sensitivity) to a range of noxious or near-noxious stimuli, most commonly being mechanical (pressure) and thermal (cold or heat) stimuli. However, the non-dermatomal nature of the condition means that sensory hyperalgesia may be identified across very different regions of the body. For example, we and others have found that people who show sensitivity to pressure pain in the uninjured tibialis anterior muscle of the lower leg after a whiplash injury are less likely to recover (Sterling, 2010; Walton et al., 2011). The working hypothesis for that phenomenon is that sensitivity to pressure pain in a region that is anatomically distant (e.g. the leg) from the region of primary injury (e.g. the neck) may be a sign of a central nociplastic driver.

Conditioned pain modulation (CPM) as a clinical test may reveal abnormalities in these patients. CPM is most often measured by the process shown in Box 9.2. Under 'normal' physiological conditions, in a system that is functioning as it should, the second application of the test stimulus *should* reveal that the patient has become less sensitive (a higher pain threshold). Accumulating evidence has now shown that in many people with chronic pain, this phenomenon either does not work at all, or in fact is reversed, where the exposure to the conditioning stimulus (e.g. cold water) then makes the person *more* sensitive to the test stimulus (e.g. pressure). The jury is still out on the mechanisms here, but it has been traditionally viewed as a proxy for the ability of the

Box 9.2 Conditioned pain modulation

1. A quantifiable response to a test stimulus is captured, such as pressure pain detection threshold in the region to be tested.

2. After the test stimulus, a conditioning stimulus is then applied. This is usually a different type of intense stimulus, such as cold water immersion, electrical stimulation, or ischemic pain through sustained contraction or blood pressure cuff inflation. This needs to be at an intensity that is at or near pain tolerance.

3. After the conditioning stimulus is removed, wait a period of time (at least 30 seconds), and then re-evaluate the quantified test stimulus. While a threshold of 'normal' has not yet been firmly established, most commonly a change in pain sensitivity (an increase in pain threshold) of at least 10% from the baseline should be observed to be confident that the pain modulation system is functioning.

central nervous system to modulate incoming nociceptive signals, likely through activation of descending pathways that rev up those inhibitory interneurons – a phenomenon termed *descending nociceptive inhibitory drive* or DNIC. Spinal cord disinhibition is thought to be one mechanism associated with centrally maintained or facilitated pain, and CPM is a method that could be used to identify that. For interest's sake there are several different protocols for testing CPM, but in our lab we use a digital algometer for pressure pain detection threshold, then immersion of the hand up to the wrist in a circulating ice water bath of 3-4°C until the intensity of pain rates an 8/10, or 90 seconds have elapsed (whichever comes first), then remove the hand from the water, wait 30 seconds and retest the pressure pain detection threshold (Fig. 9.3A–C). As far as we know there has yet to be an 'acceptable' threshold on this type of test, but recent testing in our lab shows an average of about a 10% increase after cold water immersion in a sample of 50 otherwise healthy people. However, as with all such sources of evidence in this book, this test cannot be used in isolation. That is, even

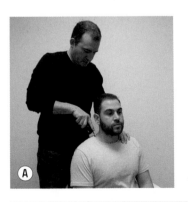 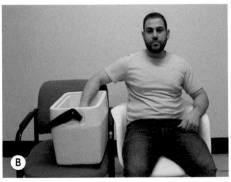 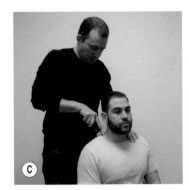

Figure 9.3A–C

An approach to evaluation of conditioned pain modulation (descending nociceptive control). (**A**) A quantifiable test stimulus is applied to the region to be tested; in this case the test stimulus is pressure pain detection threshold. (**B**) Then a conditioning stimulus is introduced that should be intense but distinct from the test stimulus. In this case the conditioning is immersion of the hand to the wrist in 3°C water for 90 seconds or until the pain reaches 8/10 intensity (whichever is first). (**C**) On removing and drying the hand, wait 30 seconds, and retest the test stimulus. A 'normal' response would be an increase in PPDT, indicating less nociceptive sensitivity.

in our healthy participants, 20–25% of them actually reported a decrease in their pain threshold (became more sensitive) following the cold water immersion, hence the value of triangulation. Another approach to this type of test would be to replace the cold water immersion with fairly intense exercise, such as a wall squat, stationary cycle, or supine chin tuck/head lift to near exhaustion (8/10 on a perceived exertion scale) and again retest with the testing stimulus (Fig. 9.4). As with the cold water, most people will show reduced sensitivity to the second test stimulus (increased threshold) after the activity, but an increasing number of researchers have now identified a subgroup of people with chronic pain that respond in the opposite way, where activity makes them *quantifiably* more sensitive to pain. This phenomenon, often referred to as 'exercise-induced hyperalgesia' is thought to be another indicator that the central sensory nociceptive processing system is not functioning properly.

Non-mechanical patterns of symptoms, including easing and aggravation, is another hallmark sign of this

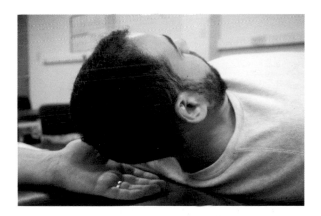

Figure 9.4
Different conditioning stimuli can be used, including ischemic compression with a blood pressure cuff, intense exercise, or isometric muscle contractions to near exhaustion. Here an alternative is shown, using isometric chin tuck/head lift for 90 seconds or until 8/10 exertion as the conditioning stimulus.

type of driver. These may be patients for whom 'every movement hurts' and 'nothing seems to relieve the pain'. There will also likely be no obvious or consistent time-based variation in the experience of pain, distinguishing it from a primary nociceptive driver that is often associated with increased pain in the morning or after a long period of inactivity but is made better with movement. Because of the potential association with immune activity, central pain may also worsen during periods of systemic illness such as a cold or flu, or in women with dysmenorrhea.

Traditional pharmaceutical approaches to pain management are unlikely to be very effective for pain driven by this domain, such as NSAIDs or other non-opioid analgesics. Opioids may be of some benefit here, as may be those same medications used in neuropathic pain (antispasmodics or antidepressants) though effectiveness of these tends to vary widely.

It is also prudent at this time to identify the overlap between this central nociplastic domain and the sensorimotor dysintegration domain that is forthcoming. In subsequent iterations of this framework, we may decide to incorporate the sensorimotor domain under this central one as the mechanisms are very similar, however for now we are keeping them separate. This is partly because this is already a heady section and for those readers new to the field of pain assessment, trying to add on the sensorimotor piece would very likely become quickly overwhelming. Further, the distinction will have implications for intervention which will become obvious later on. Having said that, some of the more unique and innovative ways of tapping sensorimotor integration will certainly add descriptive value to this nociplastic domain. These include laterality recognition, two-point discrimination, perception of body boundaries, and perhaps joint position sense.

Another bit of overlap that needs to be highlighted between this central domain and the peripheral

	Suggested evidence for triangulation: nociplastic domain	

Test domains	Findings	Shift in likelihood
Screening tools	While not as valuable here, there are some tools that have been designed to identify pain of a likely central origin. The most recognizable is the Central Sensitization Inventory (Mayer et al., 2012). The full-form of the McGill Pain Questionnaire may also have value in identifying this driver, and a new tool created by our group called the MultiDimensional Symptom Index provides subscale scores on both somatic and non-somatic (central) domains. As there is no gold standard for a central nociplastic driver of pain, the validity of such tools will always be in question.	+
Symptom behavior	Not predictable, inconsistent, no clearly mechanical pattern. Non-dermatomal or non-anatomic pain is usually present outside of any 'normal' anatomical distribution of a peripheral nerve or a single spinal dermatome. Mirror pain that spreads from one side to the other. Pain is often diffuse and poorly localized, could be described as sharp or dull, heavy or achy. A sense of fullness or swelling of the affected region, or a sense that the affected region is somehow not part of the patient's body may also be clues.	+++
Palpation	Unlikely to find a single muscle with tender or trigger points, though they may be present and widespread. The nature of this driver is such that no single 'tissue at fault' will be identifiable. Widespread tenderness to palpation without an obvious anatomical pattern is more likely.	+
Quantitative sensory testing	Widespread sensory hypersensitivity beyond the boundaries of a normal nerve innervation or muscle. Most common are mechanical and thermal pain stimuli in the clinic. Conditioned pain modulation (CPM) may be ineffective or even reversed. Exercise-induced hyperalgesia may be present.	++
Sensorimotor testing	Two-point discrimination, laterality recognition, joint position sense error or general proprioception may all be abnormal.	+
Mechanical testing	'Standard' clinical diagnostic tests are likely to be inconclusive. This includes orthopedic special tests as well as routine diagnostic imaging.	++
Cognitions	While not a means to identify a nociplastic driver, it should be expected that there will be strong signs of negative cognitions and psychological distress in these patients regardless of the tool chosen. These should however not be assumed to be irrational but areas for further exploration.	Neutral
Emotions	As per cognitions, adverse psychological profiles are expected but not required to endorse a central nociplastic driver.	Neutral
Socioenvironmental	Potentially interesting, but also difficult to interpret, evidence here. On balance, females tend to be more heavily represented across *most* chronic pain conditions compared to males. If many chronic pain conditions have a component of central nociplasticity, which appears likely, then one *may* argue central pain modulation may differ in effectiveness between sexes, a suggestion that has at least *some* empirical support (Martel et al., 2013). Similarly, there is evidence that, for example, there are racial and ethnic differences in vulnerability to poor central pain modulation (Mechlin et al., 2005; 2011). However, we argue that these types of findings provide at best an incomplete picture of a very complicated topic. While there may be genetic and socioenvironmental influences on the likelihood of central nociplastic change with pain, none of that evidence is at the point where we feel comfortable endorsing it for clinical use.	Neutral

Test domains	Findings	Shift in likelihood
	Suggested evidence for triangulation: nociplastic domain *continued*	
Pathology	It is expected that there will be no obvious lesion on diagnostic imaging that can explain pain with a central nociplastic driver. There is some evidence that those who experience trauma in the presence of pre-existing comorbidities such as depression or chronic stress may be more vulnerable to central change, but again much of this is in its infancy or theoretical stage. The *lack* of a clear pathomechanical lesion is the 'positive' indicator here.	+

neuropathic domain in terms of presenting signs and symptoms is allodynia. Heightened sensitivity and pain in response to normally non-painful stimuli may be a characteristic of both drivers, as may be temporal ('wind-up') and spatial summation tests. And finally, some readers may wonder how, if at all, things like stress-induced hyper- or hypoalgesia or other psychosomatic phenomena fit here (like when you become more or less sensitive to pain in response to stressful situations). While arguably systemic events, likely driven by endocrine or autonomic activity, they do not fit well in this domain focused on *plastic change of the central nervous system*. We will pick these up again in the more psychologically oriented domains. This overlap is not problematic, rather it highlights two important phenomena worth mentioning again: 1) that the experience of pain is complex and multidimensional and that it cannot nor should not be reduced to a single driver; and 2) that the concept of triangulation holds that you do not make a call on the drivers of a patient's pain experience based only on a single piece of evidence.

Prognostic value

There is consistent, and growing, evidence that those who demonstrate signs or symptoms of central nociplastic change early following an acute onset of pain are at greater risk of transitioning to chronic pain, though many of the mechanisms are currently unclear. For example, following acute whiplash associated disorder, we and others have found that those who show signs consistent with widespread sensory hypersensitivity, most commonly identified through reduced pressure pain detection thresholds at sites remote from the neck (e.g. tibialis anterior) also earn membership to the 'high-risk' group (Walton et al., 2011). Additionally, early signs of cold hypersensitivity (see Fig. 8.4), appear to earn people membership to the group more likely to continue to report pain six or twelve months later. Similar findings have been reported for acute low back pain (this time the 'remote' site is the forearm) (Starkweather et al., 2016). Kim and colleagues used the Central Sensitization Inventory to group people with osteoarthritis undergoing total knee joint arthroplasty into "likely" or "not likely" central sensitivity. The *likely central sensitivity* group had worse postoperative outcomes immediately and at one and three month follow-ups, and required more rescue medication (Kim et al., 2015). These are just examples – similar findings have been reported for headache pain, temporomandibular disorders, and upper extremity 'overuse' disorders. The evidence is fairly consistent so far: inasmuch as central nociplasticity can be confidently identified, those who demonstrate this as a strong driver of their acute pain experience are more likely to report persistent pain and other poor outcomes at follow-up, regardless of the body region affected.

Intervention strategies

This is one of the more difficult drivers for which empirical evidence can be found to support clinical decisions, partly because the diagnostic criteria remain unclear. There is some evidence that the same pharmaceutical approaches used for neuropathic pain, including gabapentin, pregabalin, SSRIs and tricyclic antidepressants, *may* have benefit in at least a subgroup of the population with a strong central driver. Implantable spinal cord stimulators have been used and found effective in some people with so-called 'failed back surgery syndrome', and transcranial magnetic stimulation (TMS) especially of the motor cortex may have value in some people with intractable chronic pain. Using complex regional pain syndrome (CRPS) or phantom limb pain (PLP) as a model for central nociplastic drivers, some clinicians have found success using motor imagery, hand laterality recognition, and mirror box therapy (in that order) as a means to 'turn down' the sensitivity (Moseley, 2004). In the absence of strong evidence, clinicians should not be afraid to lean on their clinical reasoning and creativity, however.

Unlike the nociceptive domain, clinicians should not expect to find a biomechanical dysfunction or structural/soft tissue lesion that can be addressed easily through mobilization or exercise, but both such approaches may still have value. Special attention should however be given to the possibility of exercise-induced hyperalgesia, meaning that not every patient with a central nociplastic driver should be expected to benefit from exercise.

For success in this domain, clinicians need to switch the way they conceptualize pain, from tissues or joints that are not functioning 'properly' (whatever that means), to a nervous system that has turned its sensitivity to *any* stimuli way up. A useful analogy that we like is the concept of a 'buffer zone' (Fig. 9.5). If we imagine a normally-functioning threat detection system, it should work such that we are alerted to potential harm and mobilize 'escape' or 'protect' resources *just before* actual tissue damage occurs. So, I stand in bare feet on hot asphalt in the summer, I should be alerted to the likelihood of impending damage just before I actually burn the bottom of my feet, giving

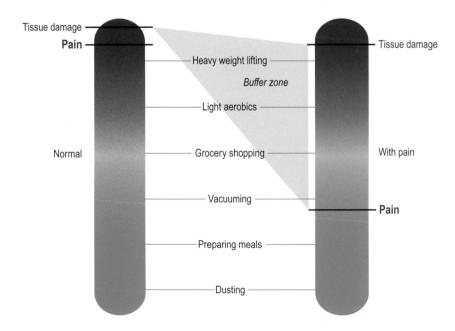

Figure 9.5
The amplified pain processing system in a hyperalgesic nervous system. If these thermometers represent amplitude of tissue stress with different activities, under normal conditions a small buffer zone should alert you to potential tissue harm or damage just before tissues actually pass their failure point. Under hyperalgesic conditions, while the tolerance of the tissues may be impaired slightly, the biggest effect is the much larger buffer zone. Now, the tissue damage warning is triggered at far lower tissue tension activities.

me a split second to voluntarily (or reflexively) lift my feet and find a cooler surface. In the case of a centrally sensitized system, that warning system, what we're calling the buffer zone between alarm and actual damage, has increased dramatically. To expand our analogy, in this case even an otherwise comfortably warm surface may be perceived as threatening, and trigger a pain experience, despite the thermal 'threat' being not intense enough to cause actual damage.

Recognizing the value of analogy, another way of thinking about a sensitized threat detection system is to consider an old house. Some readers may live in a house that tends to creak and groan at night, especially as the outside temperature cools and the materials in your house naturally expand and contract. If you've lived there for a while you likely don't think too much about the creaks and groans. Now let's imagine that you return home one night to find your old house has been broken into and many valuable items have been stolen. Having had your personal sanctity violated, you now become hypervigilant to *any* potential signs of impending danger. Those very same creaks and groans now could be interpreted as footsteps on a staircase and keep you up at night. Same stimuli, very different experience owing to a prior threat to your safety and security.

So, if the central nociplastic domain can be conceptualized as a central nervous system that is hypervigilant towards any potential threat cues, then intervention should be provided from that perspective. Exercise or activity-based interventions should not be prescribed from the viewpoint of lengthening or strengthening tissues (though that may be a nice side effect), but rather from the perspective of trying to 'retrain' a hair-trigger alarm system. Find activities or movements that you think will bring the nervous system *near* the point 'Alarm! Threat! Pain!' but not *through* it. Imagine that you're retraining the system to let it know 'this is ok, this movement is safe, no

need for alarm here'. It's a tender point to reach and requires a bit of trial and error – if you do go through the alarm threshold, it's possible you've undone much of your work and the system sensitizes again. This is admittedly hypothetical but has been a useful framework in our own clinical experiences. This can also be a good time to open discussion with your patient that hurt and harm are not the same thing – tapping into the cognitive domain that we'll address in Chapter 10.

Using the notion of 'up to but not beyond' and introducing novel, non-threatening stimuli to a sensitized system, you can start to create different approaches to health and wellness by helping your patient with a strong central nociplastic driver and using the various tools in your own toolbox. Touch can be very powerful, and considerable work in rats has shown that physical contact leads to creation of new neuronal synapses or modification of existing ones, so perhaps manual contact of painful body regions can also induce beneficial neural changes in humans. We've already mentioned graded activity and exercise, motor imagery, laterality recognition, and mirror box therapy, in addition to pharmacotherapy and perhaps cognitive reframing of painful experiences. There are several other potential options here, including electrophysical agents, needling, mindfulness-based movement (e.g. Feldenkrais method) or meditation approaches. However, caution is urged here because we could simply be opening the opportunity for any provider to undertake any intervention under the auspices of 'this might work'. Here, we will lean back on one of our favorite sayings, that *everything will work for someone, but nothing works for everyone*. If you start down this path following the APT framework, then you've already collected a series of metrics that can be used to evaluate change over time. The challenge for clinicians is to try to match the right treatment to the right person at the right time, and systematic use of standardized outcome measures will help you know if you're on the right track or if you need to abandon one direction in favor of another. Be thoughtful, prudent, and judicious in your clinical approach to people with a strong nociplastic driver and we are confident that you will be able to help a large proportion of this population.

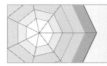

Case study
Central nociplastic domain findings

There is some evidence from Sean's case so far that there is a component of his pain experience that is being driven more by the central nociceptive (pain) processing pathways than the peripheral tissue injury, though so far, it is quite unclear. On the 'supporting' side are the not-quite-consistent movement based findings where every motion hurts (though some more than others), a considerable prior history of neck pain and headaches, and the symptoms he describes related to difficulties with concentration and eye fatigue, though in the absence of a clear *pain* contribution these probably fit better with sensorimotor than nociceptive central processing

problems. On the 'refuting' side, the onset is fairly acute, we did not find evidence of widespread mechanical hypersensitivity on pressure pain detection threshold testing, and his description of the pain being within a fairly localized region is consistent with the mechanism of injury. We also like that his pain does seem to fluctuate (based on the BPI pain severity scores from our go-to toolbox), but none of these are strong enough indicators to tell us we can ignore a central nociplastic driver.

For additional triangulation we have several options. We *could* have him complete a self-report tool such as the Central Sensitization Inventory, though for pain-related problems the CSI can be difficult to interpret. Since we've already captured his pressure pain detection threshold (PPDT), however, we can use that as a baseline for a test of conditioned pain modulation. In choosing a 'conditioning' stimulus, we need a different modality for causing an intense and unpleasant experience than mechanical pressure. We could have Sean immerse his hand in a bucket of ice water for up to 90 seconds if one were available, but in the absence of that we'll use an isometric muscle test to induce anaerobic-type pain. Since we know his lower extremities have not

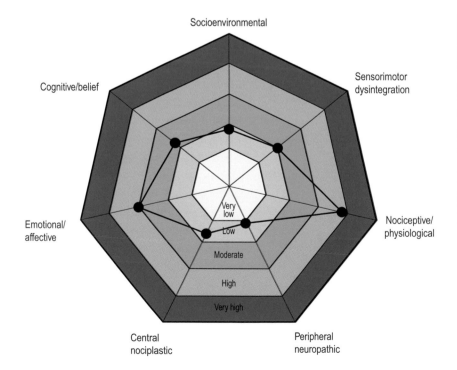

Figure 9.6
Sean's radar plot continues to take shape. Based on the central nociplastic domain findings, this driver has been kept at 'low' probability.

been affected, an isometric wall squat will work here. Sean is asked to stand with his back against a wall and squat down until his knees are flexed 90 degrees then hold that position as long as possible. Ideally, we want to hit an 8 or 9 out of 10 on a perceived exertion scale (some readers may be familiar with a Borg scale for this purpose), so just before he collapses from exhaustion. For most people that will be around 90-120 seconds, though outliers do exist. Sean manages to hold the squat for a full 2 minutes after which he sits again, red faced but not otherwise harmed. After 30 seconds we retest the PPDT about the left neck, and his pain threshold has *increased* (become less sensitive) by 20% from baseline. This indicates a normally functioning central nociceptive processing system and provides important evidence for triangulation that a central nociplastic driver is not a strong (in relative terms) contributor to his pain experience. For now, we'll label that driver in the 'low' range (Fig. 9.6). That is, we won't ignore it and may need to revisit if the symptoms persist, but for now it is not the best place for us to dedicate our intervention efforts.

References

Davis, K. D., Flor, H., Greely, H. T., et al., 2017. Brain imaging tests for chronic pain: medical, legal and ethical issues and recommendations. *Nature Reviews. Neurology* 13 (10):624–38.

Flor, H., Braun, C., Elbert, T., et al., 1997. Extensive reorganization of primary somatosensory cortex in chronic back pain patients. *Neuroscience Letters* 224 (1):5–8.

Kim, S. H., Yoon, K. B., Yoon, D. M., et al., 2015. Influence of centrally mediated symptoms on postoperative pain in osteoarthritis patients undergoing total knee arthroplasty: A prospective observational evaluation. *Pain Practice* 15 (6):E46–E53.

Kuchinad, A., Schweinhardt, P., Seminowicz, D. A., et al., 2007. Accelerated brain gray matter loss in fibromyalgia patients: premature aging of the brain? *Journal of Neuroscience* 27 (15):4004–7.

Martel, M. O., Wasan, A. D., Edwards, R. R., 2013. Sex differences in the stability of conditioned pain modulation (CPM) among patients with chronic pain. *Pain Medicine* 14 (11):1757–68.

Mayer, T. G., Neblett, R., Cohen, H., et al., 2012. The development and psychometric validation of the central sensitization inventory. *Pain Practice* 12 (4): 276–85.

Mechlin, M. B., Maixner, W., Light, K. C., et al., 2005. African Americans show alterations in endogenous pain regulatory mechanisms and reduced pain tolerance to experimental pain procedures. *Psychosomatic Medicine* 67 (6): 948–56.

Mechlin, B., Heymen, S., Edwards, C. L., et al., 2011. Ethnic differences in cardiovascular-somatosensory interactions and in the central processing of noxious stimuli. *Psychophysiology* 48 (6):762–73.

Moseley, G. L., 2004. Graded motor imagery is effective for long-standing complex regional pain syndrome: a randomised controlled trial. *Pain* 108 (1–2):192–8.

Rodriguez-Raecke, R., Niemeier, A., Ihle, K., et al., 2009. Brain gray matter decrease in chronic pain is the consequence and not the cause of pain. *Journal of Neuroscience* 29 (44):13746–50.

Seminowicz, D. A., Wideman, T. H., Naso, L., et al., 2011. Effective treatment of chronic low back pain in humans reverses abnormal brain anatomy and function. *The Journal of Neuroscience* 31 (20):7540–50.

Starkweather, A. R., Lyon, D. E., Kinser, P., et al., 2016. Comparison of low back pain recovery and persistence. *Biological Research For Nursing* 18 (4):401–10.

Sterling, M., 2010. Differential development of sensory hypersensitivity and a measure of spinal cord hyperexcitability following whiplash injury. *Pain* 150 (3):501–6.

Walton, D., Macdermid J. C., Nielson, W., et al., 2011. Pressure pain threshold testing demonstrates predictive ability in people with acute whiplash. *Journal of Orthopedic and Sports Physical Therapy* 41 (9):658–65.

10

The Cognitive Domain

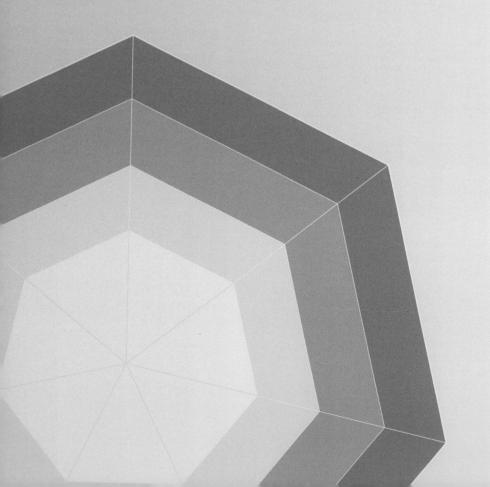

Proposed mechanisms

If the central nociplastic domain represents one of the *currently* most active areas of pain science research, the cognitive domain easily takes the crown for the *historically* most active over the past two decades or so. It's challenging to exactly pinpoint when the explosion in cognitive-behavioral research foci commenced, but the latter half of the 1990s represents a good starting-point. That said, we'd be remiss to ignore the seminal works from Dr. Gordon Waddell, where in the 1970s and 80s he proposed that non-organic signs (and fear-avoidance) were crucial to our understanding of a patient's experience with their pain. We must also recognize George Engel's initial description of the biopsychosocial model of health and wellness in 1977 (Fig. 10.1); though it wasn't immediately applied to pain. Looking to the late 1990s we can see the biopsychosocial movement for understanding pain really gaining steam, with a number of what have since become high-profile publications from 1998-2000. Ronald Melzack's *Neuromatrix Model* of pain (Fig. 10.2) and Louis Gifford's *Mature Organism Model* (Fig. 10.3) (both of which heavily featured the psyche and its role in interpreting various input and stimuli), raised our understanding of why no two tissue injuries appeared to present in the same way. A few years prior to this, in 1995, Canadian psychologist Michael Sullivan first published the increasingly popular *Pain Catastrophizing Scale*, ushering in a new era of cognition-based examinations of the patient's experience of pain. In 2000, Johan Vlaeyen and Stephen Linton published their *Fear-Avoidance Model* (FA model; Fig. 10.4) for explaining how cognitions drive the patient's transition from acute to chronic pain. The FA model has since become one of the most widely recognized explanations for why some, but not all, people develop chronic pain following an acute and distressing event.

Work in the area of cognitions, beliefs, expectations, representations, and other related constructs has continued with zest since the turn of the century. A quick search of the online peer-reviewed article database *PubMed* using the terms 'Pain Catastrophizing Scale' from inception to April 2019 reveals that there have been over 630 manuscripts published since 1995 using the Pain Catastrophizing Scale alone, with an average of about 50+ per year as of 2008. Not bad for a single scale, and for good reason: pain-related cognitions continue to be one of the most consistent predictors of current and future pain and disability across conditions and body regions.

With that context then, there is no way we can reasonably attempt to summarize all possible mechanisms that may be at play to explain the relationships between cognitions and pain, so we'll focus on the most representative ones:

1. Cognitions driving behaviors,

2. Cognitions driving physiology, and

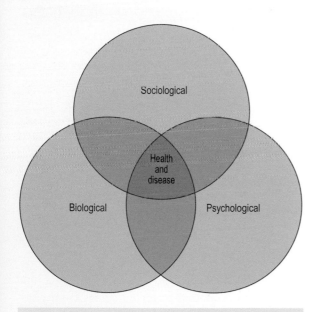

Figure 10.1
A diagrammatic representation of Engel's (1977) biopsychosocial model of health and disease. Representing a departure from the dominant biomedical model of the time, the biopsychosocial model recognized and respected that health and deviations therefrom (i.e. disease) were never fully reducible to being simply a deviation from otherwise 'normal' biological status or processes. This model has since strongly informed the World Health Organization's *International Classification of Functioning, Disability, and Health* (ICF) model that is currently the dominant model of health and disease.

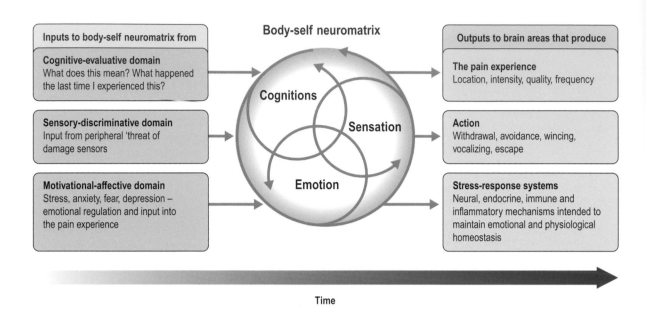

Figure 10.2

The Neuromatrix Model of Pain. This model indicates that pain is better conceived not solely as the result of nociceptive input from the periphery (that notion was tossed away with the Gate Control Theory in the 1960s) but rather as a combination of *Sensory-Discriminative* (Where in the body is this happening? How many nociceptors are activated? How widespread is it?), *Cognitive-Evaluative* (What does this mean? How dangerous is it? What happened the last time I experienced this?), and *Motivational-Affective* (What is my current mood? How does this new information make me feel? Is this something I can or want to escape from?). Only when all three of those domains are in agreement that this experience is intense, unpleasant, could signal harm, and induces a sense of fear or avoidance/withdrawal, will pain be the output. Notably, the Neuromatrix Model also provided an opportunity to adopt some consistent language around describing the nature of pain as an output, in that pain could be *described* in terms of perceptual, behavioral (actions), and coping (stress regulation) domains. (Adapted from Melzack, R., 1999. From the gate to the neuromatrix. *Pain* Suppl 6:S121–6.).

3. The complicated connection between self-report tools for measuring cognitions and those for measuring pain.

Self-report tools for measuring cognitions and pain

We'll start with the last one first and hearken back to the last sentence of the prior paragraph: that pain-related cognitions *continue to be one of the most consistent predictors of current and future pain and disability across conditions and body regions*. This appears to be the case in neck, low back, shoulder, knee, elbow, headache, and temporomandibular and orofacial pain, as well as for outcomes from pharmaceutical management, surgery, and conservative rehabilitation. Those patients who score high on a scale asking about: a) how terrible is the experience of pain; b) how well they feel they are in control; or c) how negatively they expect their outcomes to be, will consistently score high (worse) on scales asking about pain and functional interference. And while this is probably more speculative than easily testable, that last statement should alert you to something: both pain and cognitions are necessarily measured

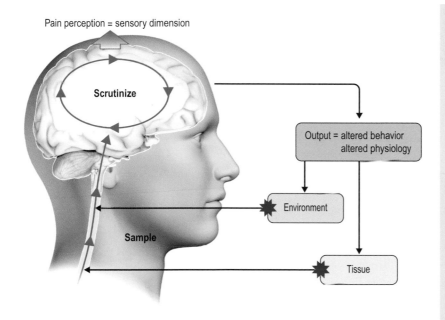

Figure 10.3
The Mature Organism Model. Similar to the Neuromatrix Model, Gifford's model respected the strong influences of meaning, past experiences and available coping resources in the interpretation and perception of nociception into pain. Gifford's model, us described in his seminal 1998 paper, also described how each experience of pain then feeds back into the memory archive that then influences subsequent experiences of pain. (Adapted with permission from Gifford, L., 1998. Pain, the tissues and the nervous system: A conceptual model. *Physiotherapy* 84 (1):27–36. Copyright © 1998 Chartered Society of Physiotherapy. Published by Elsevier Ltd.)

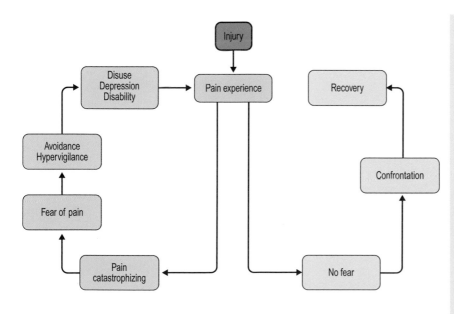

Figure 10.4
The Fear-Avoidance Model details how an individual may develop and report chronic pain resulting in behavior that resembles pain-related fear. In the acute stage, avoidant behavior can be reinforced if it results in less pain or discomfort, which could reinforce long-term avoidance of certain activities believed to increase one's pain perception. On the contrary, if the individual perceives the pain as nonthreatening or temporary, he or she feels less anxious and confronts the pain-related situation. (Adapted from Vlaeyen & Linton, 2000.)

through patient self-report, usually using some kind of standardized form. As such, it should come as no surprise that people who circle higher numbers on one form are also more likely to circle higher numbers on another, especially when both are asking questions related to the intensity or terribleness of their situation. Now, we fully recognize we may be guilty of offering a slightly cynical view on measuring a highly complex problem and equally complicated topic, but it is a general truism in research that capturing data through one mode (e.g. patient self-report) is likely to lead to better predictive models when the thing to be predicted is *also* captured through the same mode. In fact, this may (and likely is) at least one part of the explanation for why cognitions have been consistently such strong predictors of concurrent or future pain and disability, more than, say, imaging findings, quantitative sensory tests, or clinical observations. These ideas will be explored again in the prognosis section of this chapter.

Cognitions driving behavior

The *cognitions driving behavior* theory is likely the most recognizable potential mechanism underlying future pain and disability, forming the central crux of the Fear-Avoidance model. In this theory, exaggerated negative orientations towards pain or activity (commonly defined using constructs like catastrophizing, kinesiophobia, or fear-avoidance), contribute (or even lead) to people with pain withdrawing from normal social behavior or avoiding activity altogether. One cannot help but hypothesize that such behavior(s) could lead to inactivity and disuse and even worse overall health and cognitions. In fact, disuse, along with disability and depression (perhaps from social isolation when recreational activities are avoided), are the cornerstones of the FA model. In a sort of vicious cycle, the model posits that strain on tissues that have

been weakened from disuse, the emotional strain of depression, and a sense of inability to perform activities then feeds back into the experience (or at least the reporting) of pain, and the cycle continues (see Fig. 10.4).

Interestingly, despite the obvious biological connections, the disuse part of the FA model has not been consistently supported. In fact, a 2007 study of people with acute low back pain followed for up to one year revealed that, even in those who continued to report persistent (or chronic) pain, there was no clear evidence of physical deconditioning despite reduced overall daily activity (Bousema et al., 2007). In a subsequent study, Wideman and colleagues explored the sequential or 'cyclical' nature of the FA model and also found that the model only partly held up to statistical scrutiny (Wideman et al., 2009). They were unable to identify a direct causal pathway between early catastrophizing and late pain. On the contrary, they found these relationships may be more reciprocal, feeding forward and backward into each other rather than sequentially as the model proposes. They also found the depression part of that cornerstone piece did not appear to predict return to work, further supporting our position that a patient's pain is multi-factorial, never to be measured in isolation and management never to be informed from one measure.

There are also several studies supporting the FA model, but those focusing on participants in the acute stage of injury are surprisingly hard to find. In one example, a group of Swedish researchers found the cognitive construct of 'pain avoidance', measured through another scale called the *Psychological Inflexibility in Pain Scale*, predicted disability and depression three years later in a group of people with whiplash-associated disorder. This group also reported that lower educational level contributed to

There are consistent links between negative cognitions and poor pain outcomes, though causation has yet to be convincingly demonstrated. That is, do negative cognitions *cause* poor pain outcomes, or do poor pain outcomes *cause* negative cognitions? Certainly, common sense tells us either could be true.

Sir Austin Bradford Hill provided a set of criteria in 1965 that need to be satisfied before a causal relationship can be said to exist with confidence. While they have been tweaked and revised over the years, the originals are still generally recognized. They are:

1. Strength: the magnitude of effect (association or difference) should be strong enough to convince you that a relationship exists.

2. Consistency: the association should be observed and largely stable across populations, contexts, and studies.

3. Specificity: causation is easier to prove if there is a very specific site or disease process associated with a specific cause. Generic associations are easy to find, but are less likely to be causal in nature.

4. Temporality: the cause should *always* precede the effect.

5. Dose-effect: the greater the magnitude of cause, the greater should be the effect.

6. Biologic plausibility: the causal relationship should make sense based on existing knowledge.

7. Coherence: a lesser used criterion, Bradford Hill stated that the confidence in cause-and-effect is strengthened when laboratory (basic) and clinical or epidemiological evidence are consistent.

8. Experiment and Analogy: lesser used criteria; experiment refers to occasional value of simply relying on experimental evidence, where analogy refers to the consistency of effect when similar (analogous) causes or effects are used.

9. Reversibility: a later addition that we quite like in most cases, referring to the phenomenon where in a true cause-and-effect relationship, if you remove the cause, the effect should similarly reduce.

the prediction of the same outcomes, a potentially interesting story that we tie together in Chapter 12 (socioenvironmental drivers). In general, we feel confident in saying the relationships between negative cognitions and pain and disability are not likely as simple as the FA model proposes, though several of the factors in that model do seem to have at least some relationship with the likelihood of a smooth recovery and the intensity of the pain experience, hence earning a position for 'cognitions/beliefs' on the radar plot. The mechanisms are likely far more complex than any linear process can capture and include the interaction of several factors (e.g. education, genetics, and social stressors).

Cognitions driving physiology

Then we have the *cognitions driving physiology* story. Again, the pathways here are complex and interactive, and to understand the full story will likely require us to consider things like genetics (or even epigenetics), early life adversities, peri-traumatic life stressors, the microbiome, the number, and possibly the type, of pathologies on imaging, pre-existing health, and likely any number of other physiological processes. To keep things simple for this story, we'll focus more on the way exaggerated negative cognitions, fears, or expectations can influence stress system activity and hence sensitivity to noxious stimuli or the person's pain experience. If cognitions are conceptualized as the way you make sense of your experiences, the thoughts that keep you up at night, or the things that influence the way you respond to life adversities, then it should not be a hard thread to draw between negative thoughts and physiological distress.

In the pain field, this represents a more recent advancement in thinking and research, and a welcome one from our perspectives. Here, the theory is that the numbers a patient circles on a form may well indicate their beliefs about their condition. But it could also provide a glimpse into the likely state of their 'fight, flight, or freeze' physiology. Arguably the most easily recognizable player in this game is cortisol, the primary stress hormone in humans and the end result of activity in the stress pathway called the *hypothalamic-pituitary-adrenal (HPA) axis* (Fig. 10.5). The hypothalamus is one of our primary control centers for ensuring that all is normal in our bodies. It is a primary player in maintaining our natural *homeostasis,* that being the relative balance between physiological processes intended to keep things within some range of 'normal'. Body temperature dropping? Hypothalamus says shiver! Blood glucose too high? Release insulin! Something threatening our very survival or well-being? Fire up the HPA! Cortisol has several wide-ranging functions depending on the target tissues it lands upon. These include mobilization of glycogen stores to provide power to muscles, redirecting blood flow so that muscles can contract and major organs are protected while things like digestion and advanced executive functions can be put on hold for a bit, mobilizing your immune and inflammatory resources to fight infection, and generally getting your body ready for maximum defense or escape functions. Of course, threats can come in different forms, including cognitions (worry, fear, catastrophic thoughts). In the cognitions driving physiology hypothesis then, it is those negative cognitions that lead to a disproportionately strong HPA drive and stress reaction, in turn driving chronic cortisol release and often reduced affinity of cortisol receptors, that may have a role in maintaining pain. While cortisol appears to have *hypo*algesic (less pain) effects in the short term (making you less aware of damage but more able to escape), prolonged systemic cortisol release appears to be associated with *hyper*algesia (more pain), possibly through some cellular cascade that leads to hypersensitized peripheral or central neurons. Effects of chronic hypercortisolism include many of the signs and symptoms we associate with chronic pain, including digestive problems, impairments in higher

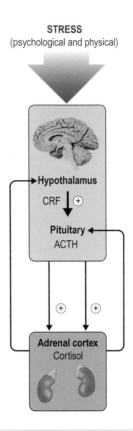

STRESS
(psychological and physical)

Figure 10.5
Diagrammatic representation of the hypothalamic-pituitary-adrenal axis. Stress or threat to the organism (whether physical or psychological) is identified by the hypothalamus as a deviation from homeostasis. Stimulation of the hypothalamus leads to the release of *corticotropin releasing factor* (CRF) that stimulates the nearby pituitary gland to release *adrenocorticotropin hormone* (ACTH) into the blood stream. As it reaches the adrenal glands on the top of the kidneys, ACTH stimulates the release of cortisol into the blood stream. Glucocorticoid (cortisol) receptors are widespread on many tissues throughout the body and can have different effects dependent on the tissue. These include mobilizing reserve energy stores in muscles (glycogen), constricting gut capillaries thereby slowing digestion, dilating vessels to the musculoskeletal system, heightening some survival senses (sight, smell, hearing) while dulling some nociceptive processes, and ultimately working its way back to the hypothalamus and pituitary to let those centers know the 'job is done' and that they can shut off further release of stimulating hormones. This is referred to as a *negative feedback loop,* and when it works properly is an incredible example of the tremendous resilience and adaptability of the human body.

order executive functions, sleep disturbances, muscle atrophy, and widespread pain itself, making this an attractive model for understanding the relationship between stress and pain.

The HPA axis is just one example of a threat-reaction pathway in humans; others that are likely equally germane to this discussion would be the sympathetic nervous system (with end products of noradrenaline/norepinephrine) and the gut-brain axis, another possible explanation for digestive problems when under chronic duress (cue, irritable bowel syndrome).

Common to all of these within the current context is that the 'stressor' or threat being detected is in the form of exaggerated negative, sometimes called 'maladaptive', cognitions that prevent the person from returning to their state of relative homeostasis. The term 'maladaptive' is intended to refer to a response to a stressor that may well be intended to cope with distress, but is, in the long run, not healthy for the organism. Perhaps this is what Melzack and Loeser were thinking of when they defined chronic pain not by duration but rather as "the inability of the body to restore its physiological functions to normal homeostatic levels" (Loeser & Melzack, 1999).

We have presented three potentially different mechanisms through which cognitions may affect pain, none of which are perfect, all of which have yet to be fully supported, and as with many such phenomena, will all likely contribute to the 'actual reality' of the matter that lies somewhere in combination of all three. As mentioned earlier, this work continues and will no doubt lead to new discoveries in the very near future. We have not delved into the influence of genetics or other life experiences on the ways cognitions and pain likely interact, and we're confident that the ongoing work towards neural networks and other 'big data' analytic techniques will provide

entirely new insights into what these complex interactions look like. For now, we hope this is enough to give you a sense of how cognitions may influence the patient's experience, or reporting, of their pain and disability.

Distinguishing features

Pain strongly driven by maladaptive cognitions is most readily identifiable through either patient narrative (the words and phrases the patient uses) or use of standardized and adequately validated patient self-report tools. This can be a difficult domain to identify because it requires the clinician to be able to distinguish between cognitions that are truly maladaptive or irrational, and those that are perfectly rational given the context of the patient. For example, a patient may state (or highly endorse the item on the Tampa Scale for Kinesiophobia) that 'pain lets me know when to stop exercising so I don't hurt myself'. Presumably this item is included on the TSK because it *may* be useful to identify those with exaggerated or irrational negative orientations towards exercise, but of course it *may* also be perfectly reasonable. For example, we neither suffer from chronic pain nor do we believe we are 'kinesiophobic', but, if we feel a strange unexpected twinge while lifting weights, we could also say that pain lets us know when to stop exercising so we don't hurt ourselves. Similarly, people with complex regional pain syndrome or phantom limb pain should be expected to score quite high on a pain-related catastrophizing scale, not necessarily because they are 'catastrophizers', but because, quite justifiably, they do in fact feel overwhelmed by the pain. They may be concerned the pain will never get any better, and in some extreme cases, may well feel that they legitimately cannot go on living like this. Are these responses irrational or are they perfectly rational given the context? Regardless, they require follow-up by the clinician for further exploration.

Chapter 10

An **important side note** with regards to knowing your questionnaire: if you're going to use the PCS, recognize that item No. 2 indicating 'I feel I can't go on' should really be followed up for possibility of suicidal ideation.

A key thing to avoid when using tools to tap the cognitive domain is to simply ascribe 'wrong thinking' to every patient who scores high on one of these tools. This requires a more nuanced exploration of the genesis and nature of these comments so that the clinician knows whether intervention should be aimed at, for example, cognitive restructuring *or* effective pain control as a first priority. Another consideration here is that we are clearly getting into territory that can be awfully close to malingering or intentional exaggeration of pain. Any time that the patient's report or narrative is considered the gold standard, we are susceptible to those who are attempting to abuse compensation or litigation processes for personal gain. Not surprisingly, opinions and values in this domain are split and, from our own experience, can become somewhat emotional at times; for both the patient and clinician. Ultimately, you should make up your own mind on where you choose to fall on issues pertaining to the likelihood of malingering in pain. For those interested, drawing upon our own clinical and research experience, we believe that: a) it is extremely difficult and taxing for any patient to maintain a façade of disability for the length of time it takes to get a case settled and that in most cases people know that it is not worth doing so; and b) short of a patient looking you in the eye and saying 'I was faking the whole time!', we believe it is nearly impossible to accurately identify the patient who is brilliantly navigating a pathway consistent with malingering behavior. Some may see our perspective as a naïve, if not biased, position. Fair enough, but to those people, we pose these questions for reflection: What do you win if you correctly identify a malingering patient? And, how many others with legitimate problems have you had to alienate to find that one? Even for those who might endorse something like Waddell's signs to identify intentional exaggeration, we urge caution. Dr. Waddell never intended his non-organic signs platform to be used for identifying the malingering patient. He developed and promoted non-organic signs to indicate a patient that may likely receive little, if any, benefit from a more invasive surgical procedure. The former position was created through misinterpretation and dare we say, has had a profound influence (negative as it may be) on the patient looking for answers for his/her persistent signs/symptoms that are not easily quantifiable with available tests and measures.

We hold the perspective that if we were to choose a position here, either to: a) doubt everyone with unexplainable chronic pain and assume all are malingerers; or to b) believe everyone and assume none are malingerers, eventually we're going to make a mistake. In the former, that mistake means that we will avoid getting tricked by those very few who are intentionally feigning or exaggerating but will also have withheld treatment from some people who truly needed it. In the latter, that mistake means we will have provided treatment to someone who didn't really need it, but will have also never failed to provide necessary treatment to those who did. When viewed from that perspective there is only one of those mistakes we are willing to make.

Prognostic value

Almost all prognostic (risk screening) tools we can think of in the rehab space can best be classed as tapping cognitions. In fact, there are only two recent ones that come to mind that include anything *other* than cognitions or beliefs. One would be the Danish Whiplash Study Group Risk Assessment Score derived by Prof. Helge Kasch and his colleagues from Aarhus University in Denmark (Kasch et al., 2011). That tool includes cervical range of motion

	Suggested evidence for triangulation: cognitive domain	
Test domains	**Findings**	**Shift in likelihood**
Screening tools	This being an active research area for some time, there are several cognition-related tools now in existence. Not all are created equal though, and clinicians should use their critical thinking skills when selecting one for their patient. Some of our favorites are the Brief Illness Perceptions Survey, the Tampa Scale for Kinesiophobia, and the Pain Self-Efficacy Questionnaire. Coping strategies questionnaires would also fit here, including things like the Chronic Pain Coping Inventory and the Coping Strategies Questionnaire. We are saving psychopathology screening questionnaires for the next domain on emotional drivers, though in some ways they could still fit here (see the prognosis section of this chapter for more on this topic). While the shift in likelihood will be strong based on the results of self-report tools, we urge caution in simply assuming all such scores indicate irrational or maladaptive beliefs. See above for a more fulsome discussion on this point.	+++
Symptom behavior	Those with a strong cognitive driver are likely to also interpret any uncomfortable sensation as potentially threatening and painful. As such, especially in the absence of a strong nociceptive driver, the clinician should expect that those with purely cognitive drivers may have slightly bizarre and inconsistent pain patterns that do not seem to conform to known anatomy or biomechanics. This is of course similar to many of the other domains of the radar plot, so the shift in confidence of a cognitive driver based solely on symptom behavior is very low.	Neutral
Palpation	Similar to symptom behavior, it is possible that palpation of any known structure is described as painful (i.e. due to fear of pain), though in the presence of a pure cognitive driver, this is unlikely to be consistent with a clear inflammatory or mechanical problem.	Neutral
Quantitative sensory testing	The general theme continues here, in that those with strong catastrophic tendencies are likely to report pain at a lower threshold than those with more adaptive cognitions, though these are unlikely to be consistent findings and will provide very little shift in likelihood (beyond the inconsistency) that cognitions are driving these findings more than other domains.	Neutral
Sensorimotor testing	As most sensorimotor tests are not intended to be pain-provoking, it is unlikely that sensorimotor testing will provide a meaningful shift in likelihood of a strong cognitive driver. The possible exception here will be those who are *so* avoidant of pain and movement that they simply are unable to reliably complete any sensorimotor test at all, though this would be rare.	Neutral
Mechanical testing	Again, the only potentially useful clue of a strong cognitive driver is that every clinical test or observation appears to illicit or worsen pain, but not in any obvious biomechanical pattern. As this is also a similar pattern in other domains such as central nociplastic drivers, these findings are of little clinical value for identifying this domain.	Neutral
Cognitions	Clearly the strongest indicator by definition, and overlapping somewhat with the screening tools item above. However, cognitions need not only be identified through standardized tools but are arguably even more readily identifiable through good questioning, patient narrative, and active listening by the clinician. Words or phrases that appear to indicate fear or concern out of proportion to the responses of most other people with a similar condition under similar demographic and cultural contexts, may be useful clues. Again, we urge caution in *assuming* that all such utterances indicate a patient who is 'thinking wrong', but they should be a clue to the clinician that a follow-up question is needed to further understand the patient's perspective on their condition.	+++

continued

	Suggested evidence for triangulation: cognitive domain *continued*	
Test domains	**Findings**	**Shift in likelihood**
Emotions	As both cognitions and emotions are part of a broader *psychological* domain, there is bound to be considerable overlap. Indeed, there is no shortage of evidence to show that, for example, scores on the Pain Catastrophizing Scale are associated with scores on depression or anxiety screening tools. The general thinking here is that maladaptive cognitions, that drive things like worry and rumination, will eventually turn into full-blown diagnosable psychopathology, so the degree to which these two domains are related likely depends at least somewhat on where in the course of the condition you see the patient. Then there are constructs such as 'anxiety sensitivity', which can be most easily conceptualized as 'catastrophizing about the symptoms of anxiety', which in turn amplifies the anxiety, and together shows just how difficult (and often unnecessary) it can be to tease these things apart.	+
	However, we do believe the distinction can be important – when we're referring to maladaptive cognitions we are NOT referring to diagnosable psychopathologies like major depressive disorder, generalized anxiety disorder, somatoform disorder, or post-traumatic stress disorder. We believe, as will be described below, that many different healthcare providers can intervene using education and thought monitoring and restructuring to address maladaptive cognitions, whereas care for people with psychopathology should really be led by a mental health professional. Nonetheless, owing to their known associations and possible causation (negative cognitions lead to emotional disorders), clinicians should expect those with a strong cognitive driver will also likely score higher on psychopathology screening tools, but how high depends on the timing and context of the interaction.	
Socioenvironmental	This domain can also be challenging, as cognitions are no doubt shaped by culture, past experiences, and broader social context. As a result, these two domains are often considered together (hence the term 'psychosocial'), though to *assume* someone is being overly negative simply because they're female, or live in poverty, or didn't finish high school, or are from a different cultural or ethnic background, would of course be inappropriate. While there is evidence to suggest that – for example, for a given experimental pain stimulus, people of African descent or females will tend to rate higher on a catastrophizing scale than those of Caucasian descent or males – it would be far too premature and misinformed to make any kind of causal attributions at this time.	Neutral
Pathology	One of the hallmarks of pain with only a strong cognitive driver will be the *absence* of clear structural lesions or pathology on diagnostic testing. In this case then, the piece of evidence is the *negative* results.	+

(more limitations in range, greater risk of non-recovery) along with other more cognitive constructs. The other would be the whiplash prognosis clinical prediction rule derived by Dr. Carrie Ritchie and colleagues in Brisbane, Australia that includes age as one of the risk variables (Ritchie et al., 2013). Other than that, every other *rehabilitation* prognostic tool we can think of measures in full or in part, cognitions, beliefs and/or expectations. These include the Traumatic Injuries Distress Scale and the STarT Back Tool. Even

in something as traditionally pathology-focused as knee osteoarthritis, a 2016 systematic review by de Rooij and colleagues found that deterioration in knee pain could best be predicted by patient reports of higher knee pain intensity, bilateral symptoms, and depressive symptoms (de Rooij et al., 2016). Other more generic tools such as the Pain Catastrophizing Scale and the Tampa Scale for Kinesiophobia, both of which are more relevant for chronic pain problems, have shown consistent ability to predict outcomes following both surgical and conservative interventions. The cognitively focused 'Work' subscale of the Fear-Avoidance Beliefs Questionnaire (FABQ), perhaps not surprisingly, has been a consistent predictor of return-to-work/work status in low back pain (Wertli et al., 2014).

An important consideration and caveat are required here and these will become even more important as we move into the next chapter on emotional drivers. We are conceptualizing anything that relies solely on the patient's self-report as 'cognitive' for this discussion. That would include pain intensity, scores on a region-specific disability scale, and even screening tools for psychopathology. Each of these, whether in whole or in part, can be conceptualized as tapping into the patient's cognitions, or the way the person thinks about and makes sense of their current situation. If the patient is the one providing the information, then it requires them to read and understand the question(s) on the form, understand and interpret the response options presented for answering, and most importantly, requires them to compare what is being asked (e.g. how bad is this pain?) against some internal frame of reference that will have been shaped over years of different experiences and outcomes. So, while we will be alluding to emotional screening tools in the next chapter on psychopathology, those tools still require the respondent (patient) to pick up a pencil or click a button and choose one answer option over another, so they cannot be disentangled from the cognitive tasks of interpretation, internal comparison, and selecting a response. In that context, true 'diagnosis' of a psychopathology should be left to a mental health professional.

Cognitions, and the tools intended to capture them, are probably *best* suited to predicting outcomes, either the clinical or natural course (or both). For most musculoskeletal conditions, these are the constructs and tools that are the most consistent predictors of outcome, including pain intensity at intake, region-specific or generic disability scores, pain-related catastrophizing, feelings or beliefs of victimization and injustice, low expectations for recovery, and fear of reinjury, among others. However, it is important to remember the caveats we presented earlier, which is that a poor outcome should not be blamed simply on the patient's 'wrong' thinking about their condition. There are several criteria that need to be satisfied before any attributions of causation (e.g. that catastrophizing *causes* chronic pain) can be made. These include things like addressing potential confounders (could there be something else influencing both cognitions *and* recovery?) and reversibility (if you specifically intervene by targeting maladaptive cognitions, recovery rates should improve, right?). Using those two as examples, the evidence for causation is not terribly compelling. For example, it could simply be the case that the reason self-reports are so good at predicting outcomes is because the outcomes being predicted are *also* patient self-reported. Both statistically and theoretically, it would make sense that the best predictor of any outcome is the same (or similar) outcome captured at intake. So, if the outcome is capturing cognitions (e.g. pain intensity, sense of disability, perceived work capacity) then the best predictors of those will also be tools capturing cognitions. Even more problematic are some recent well-designed clinical trials that explored the effectiveness of early interventions that specifically targeted maladaptive cognitions as part of the treatment plan for acute musculoskeletal trauma. So far, these strategies have not consistently demonstrated any significant improvement in outcomes for both neck (Jull et al., 2013; Lamb et al., 2013) and low back pain (Traeger et al., 2019). This is problematic for the 'cognitions camp' because, presumably, if exaggerated (maladaptive) distress, fear or catastrophizing

Chapter 10

were in fact causing the lack of recovery, then you'd think that by specifically targeting the cause you'd see some similar reduction in the effect. A recent randomized trial has shown some effectiveness of psychologically trained physiotherapist intervention for acute whiplash (Sterling et al., 2019). While the effects were generally small, the superior outcomes in the active group, for one of the first times, provide evidence that targeting intervention at cognitive risk factors may, in fact, improve outcomes, for those with identifiable cognitive risk factors.

If we were to offer a potential reason for the generally small effects of these types of treatment, it would be that we, and others, believe that whether or not someone recovers from musculoskeletal trauma is based on *more* than just the numbers they circle on a form, despite those forms and numbers being consistent predictors of outcome. Assuming the forms that patients are completing are valid measures of the intended latent construct in the first place, there are very likely *other* players involved in the likelihood of recovery – for example, perhaps heightened posttraumatic distress is only a problem when present in someone who *also* has genetic or social vulnerabilities, and all of these factors interact in complex ways to influence the likelihood and course of recovery. This is work that is ongoing around the world and exciting developments are likely to come in the near future.

Intervention strategies

Having just described some of the recent findings from clinical trials targeting maladaptive cognitions, the bulk of this discussion is going to be more theoretical in nature rather than empirical. Arguably the most important component of intervention for maladaptive cognitions is to recognize those that are indeed maladaptive and irrational. As we described earlier, in some contexts or conditions, it would be perfectly

adaptive and rational to have thoughts about feeling overwhelmed by pain, fearing re-injury, or feeling distressed about the traumatic event. In fact, we believe there could be equal alarm in seeing people who seem to have *no* reaction to pain or trauma – could they be repressing their emotions or be detached from the experience? As such, we implore clinicians to select one or two pain-related cognitions tools targeted to their population with which they can get familiar, and to use those to optimal effect. Optimal in this case means going beyond just knowing what the summed score means as far as good or bad, but also reviewing the patient's response to each individual item on the scale or form. In short, know your scale and know it well. An astute clinician should then be able to use those to frame the patient interview: 'I see you've indicated here that you expect this pain is going to last a very long time. Is that accurate? If so, can you tell me more about why you think that?' In this way, the scales or tools and the item responses *inform* the patient interview, improving it, rather than replacing it. Through use of carefully crafted questions, clinicians can start to develop a better understanding of how the patient is framing (representations for) their condition and can make more informed decisions on whether they are: a) inaccurate or irrational; and b) amenable to intervention.

Where problematic cognitions or beliefs are identified, we see options based on the values and worldviews of the patient. In some cases, a well-crafted educational intervention may be useful. However, clinicians are encouraged to reflect on what a 'well-crafted' educational intervention should look like. This is not simply handing the patient a pamphlet nor is it rote recitation of some canned set of punitive comments about why they're wrong. Like a professional primary or secondary school teacher, clinicians wishing to provide a sound educational intervention need to consider the starting knowledge, attitudes,

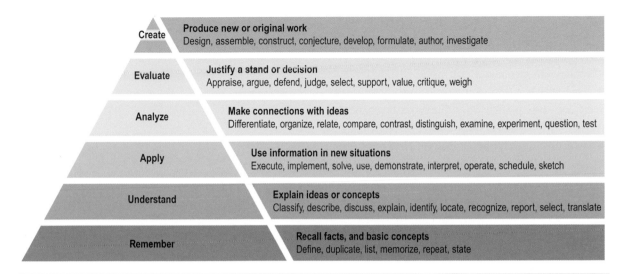

Figure 10.6

Bloom's most recent taxonomy of cognitive learning outcomes. Clinicians should keep this pyramid in mind when designing educational interventions for their patients. Where on the journey is this patient starting in terms of their understanding of pain, and where do they need to be in order for the intervention to be considered a success? In some cases, all a clinician needs is for a patient to at least understand certain concepts. For example, where there have been descriptions of patients writing their own books, short stories, poems or other works about pain, that would be at the level of creation.

and values of the patient and try to identify how they learn best. Usually this can be accomplished through direct questioning, though not everyone will know how they learn best. The clinician may wish to consult something like Bloom's Taxonomy of cognitive learning outcomes and decide which level of learning the patient needs to attain in order to be able to use the information (Fig. 10.6). Then the content needs to be created, thinking specifically about what *this* patient needs to know at *this* time. And to what end? How will you know if the educational intervention has been successful? Perhaps it is a re-evaluation using the same cognitive tool, though what constitutes meaningful change on many such tools is largely unknown.

Of course, education is not the right choice for everyone, so clinicians may need to consider other ways to address pain or mobility issues that have a strong cognitive driver. Another sound approach would be to draw from exposure-based therapies for phobias. Several such approaches have been explored in research, and by most indications, in the right people, a graded exposure or graduated activity-type approach (the latter usually requiring a more detailed plan of milestones and criteria for progression) appear to have some value. Some of the more well-recognized work in the area has come from Prof. Stephen Linton's group from Orebro University in Sweden. Prof. Linton and colleagues published a series of papers through the 2000s–2010s on 'exposure in vivo' to show generally modest effects on pain, function, and negative cognitions (Boersma et al., 2004; Linton et al., 2008). In these strategies, patients first create a customized hierarchy of 'feared movements' usually by selecting photographs of people doing different activities, then ranking them in terms of how fearful they would be to engage in those activities. The clinicians then work with the patients, starting with the first (lowest fear) activity and creatively coming up with ways to expose the patient to aspects of those activities, perhaps through imagery or observation or activities that get closer and closer to the most feared one. They then have the patient reflect on their actual pain experiences as a result. The idea here – and this is why such an approach should only be used with patients that have clear irrational beliefs – is that after having been exposed to the feared activity, the activity-related impact on their pain is not as bad as they expected, thereby challenging those fear-avoidance beliefs. It is, however, a tricky thing to get right and not everyone will want to do this (and it can backfire if not provided properly), but some of the simpler ideas, like starting low and progressing in activity or exercise intensity can be another way of targeting maladaptive beliefs.

Regardless of the strategy taken, it is important to always think about the 'why' here. Why do you believe the patient requires education? Why do you believe graded activity is a good option? Is this the right time to challenge their beliefs? These kinds of questions should form the basis for all rehabilitation interventions for pain, but perhaps none more so than for pain with a strong cognitive driver. These are also critical questions in the patient's interest, as poorly conceived or delivered education can have more of a detrimental effect than a positive one. And clinicians should avoid falling into the trap of assuming that: a) everyone *wants* to learn about pain; and b) everyone learns the same way that 'you' do.

While research appears to indicate that many interventions are unlikely to succeed until highly exaggerated negative beliefs about pain are addressed,

they do need to be approached carefully and with respect for the patient in front of you. It is here that we confidently believe such an approach may need to be delayed until a strong patient-provider alliance has been formed.

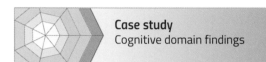

Case study
Cognitive domain findings

From our initial conversations with Sean and the results of the go-to toolbox, it is already fairly clear that this trauma has been a distressing experience. Keep in mind this does *not* mean Sean is simply weak-willed or that his thoughts and perceptions are somehow irrational or maladaptive; most people *should* experience some degree of increased emotional distress following a significant trauma (actually we'd be more concerned if his affect was completely flat). What we're trying to sort out here is the relative degree to which exaggerated negative appraisals or perceptions are contributing to his pain experience, and in turn may interfere with engagement in treatment or the effectiveness thereof.

Another goal at this stage will be to try to distinguish between misinterpretations or misappraisals and diagnosable mood disorders or psychopathology. The former can potentially be addressed by appropriately targeted educational interventions, while the latter will likely require the services of a mental health professional. In that spirit, a logical step here would be to administer an emotional disorder screening tool, such as a depression or acute stress disorder scale, and if that is negative, it would lend more support for a cognitive driver than an emotional one. Another way of stating this is to say, in the absence of a likely emotional disorder like depression (which if present at this acute stage would likely have been pre-existing rather than a result of the trauma, but could still interfere with smooth recovery), then any negative appraisals, beliefs, or perceptions can likely be addressed by an appropriately informed talk- or graded-activity type intervention.

While there are very many pain-related cognitions tools freely available, there are surprisingly few intended for use in

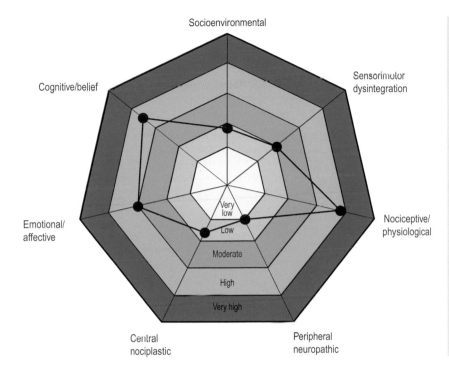

Figure 10.7
Sean's radar plot continues to take shape. Based on the cognitive domain findings, this driver has been moved to 'high' probability.

acute pain. Most have been designed and intended for use in chronic pain. One of our tools, the Traumatic Injuries Distress Scale (TIDS), was designed specifically for the purposes of use in acute post-traumatic pain such as Sean's situation. Another, the Injustice Experience Questionnaire (IEQ) is meant to measure one's belief that they have been unfairly victimized as a result of someone else's actions and may be of value here though its direct link with pain is slightly less clear. We're finding clinicians are also increasingly attempting to apply tools like the Pain Catastrophizing Scale, the Fear-Avoidance Beliefs Questionnaire, or the Tampa Scale for Kinesiophobia for these kinds of cases, though we suggest these are not

the best tools for Sean as they were not designed with acute neck pain in mind. So, for the purposes of our case, we've had Sean complete the TIDS as a means to 'quantify' the distress he's experiencing, and for use as a tool to evaluate change in that distress over time. On the overall tool he scores 16/24, which indicates considerable post-trauma distress, and scores high on each of the subscales for *Uncontrolled pain*, *Negative affect*, and *Intrusion/Hyperarousal*. For now, we're going to bump the cognitive domain up the plot a bit as a result of the available information (Fig. 10.7), but we will revisit this in light of the emotional screening tools described in the next chapter.

References

Boersma, K., Linton, S., Overmeer, T., et al., 2004. Lowering fear-avoidance and enhancing function through exposure in vivo. A multiple baseline study across six patients with back pain. *Pain* 108 (1–2):8–16.

Bousema, E. J., Verbunt, J. A., Seelen, H. A., et al., 2007. Disuse and physical deconditioning in the first year after the onset of back pain. *Pain* 130 (3):279–86.

de Rooij, M., van der Leeden, M., Heymans, M. W., et al., 2016. Prognosis of pain and physical functioning in patients with knee osteoarthritis: A systematic review and meta-analysis. *Arthritis Care & Research* 68 (4):481–92.

Jull, G., Kenardy, J., Hendrikz, J., et al., 2013. Management of acute whiplash: a randomized controlled trial of multidisciplinary stratified treatments. *Pain* 154 (9):1798–1806.

Kasch, H., Qerama, E., Kongsted, A., et al., 2011. The risk assessment score in acute whiplash injury predicts outcome and reflects biopsychosocial factors. *Spine* 36 (25 Suppl):S263–7.

Lamb, S. E., Gates, S., Williams, M. A., et al., 2013. Emergency department treatments and physiotherapy for acute whiplash: a pragmatic, two-step, randomised controlled trial. *The Lancet* 381 (9866):546–56.

Linton, S. J., Boersma, K., Jansson, M., et al., 2008. A randomized controlled trial of exposure in vivo for patients with spinal pain reporting fear of work-related activities. *European Journal of Pain* 12 (6):722–30.

Loeser, J. D., Melzack, R., 1999. Pain: an overview. *The Lancet* 353 (9164): 1607–9.

Ritchie, C., Hendrikz, J., Kenardy, J., et al., 2013. Derivation of a clinical prediction rule to identify both chronic moderate/severe disability and full recovery following whiplash injury. *Pain* 154 (10):2198–206.

Sterling, M., Smeets, R., Keijzers, G., et al., 2019. Physiotherapist-delivered stress inoculation training integrated with exercise versus physiotherapy exercise alone for acute whiplash-associated disorder (StressModex): a randomised controlled trial of a combined psychological/physical intervention. *British Journal of Sports Medicine* pii: bjsports-2018-100139. doi: 10.1136/bjsports-2018-100139. [Epub ahead of print].

Traeger, A. C., Lee, H., Hübscher, M., et al., 2019. Effect of intensive patient education vs placebo patient education on outcomes in patients with acute low back pain. *JAMA Neurology* 76 (2):161–9.

Vlaeyen, J., Linton, S., 2000. Fear-avoidance and its consequences in chronic musculoskeletal pain: a state of the art. *Pain* 85:317–32.

Wertli, M. M., Rasmussen-Barr, E., Weiser, S., et al., 2014. The role of fear avoidance beliefs as a prognostic factor for outcome in patients with nonspecific low back pain: a systematic review. *The Spine Journal* 14 (5):816–36.e4.

Wideman, T. H., Adams, H., Sullivan, M. J., 2009. A prospective sequential analysis of the fear-avoidance model of pain. *Pain* 145 (1–2):45–51.

11

The Emotional Domain

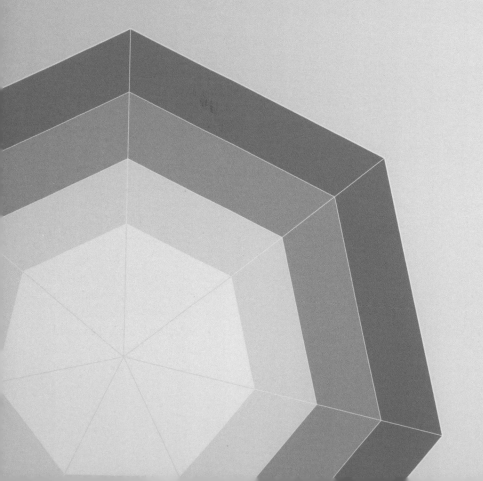

Proposed mechanisms

To begin, this chapter requires us to provide some definitions and clarifications. Many who espouse to subscribe to the 'biopsychosocial' model of pain will unknowingly reduce many pain drivers to either 'biological' or 'psychosocial'. The term *psychosocial,* as its often used, is a bit of a misnomer. Many clinicians appear to be using the term to refer to any patient's pain that cannot be clearly attributed to structural pathology, though in doing so it has almost become somewhat pejorative. 'This patient is very psychosocial' is something we've read with alarming frequency on patient charts or reports, and this appears to indicate a misunderstanding of the realities of pain (and the models thereof). First, it is important to keep in mind that the distinction between biology, psychology, and social context are largely artificial – none exists without the others. As we stated in Chapter 10, there is no psychology (a series of firing neurons and resultant behavior) without biology, and biology and psychology only exist in the ways we know of them due to the way environmental and social pressures have shaped them. But, at the same time, societies have been formed to be responsive to and accommodative of the biology and psychology of humans. So, the often-siloed approach to understanding pain though 'biological', 'psychological' and 'social' lenses, while arguably necessary (or at least facilitatory) for research and debate, is artificial and many would argue, overly reductionistic.

While we recognize and respect that any experience as complex as pain is irreducible, we also don't believe that clinicians or researchers using the term, 'psychosocial' are using it from that position. In the interest of trying to better understand the drivers of the pain experience, as we are doing with this current APT framework, we argue that the term 'psychosocial' is not only potentially harmful when used pejoratively, but also dramatically oversimplifies some fairly complex interactions. Without getting too far off track though, we're first going to at least separate the 'psycho' from the 'social', the latter of which will be the topic of Chapter 12. By combining those two broad areas of focus into a single 'psychosocial' term, we do justice to neither.

If we zoom in on the psychological domain, many people will get confused by our strategy to separate 'psycho' into two domains: a cognitive (Chapter 10) and an emotional domain (this chapter). Both cognitions and emotions are clearly related to psychology, clearly drive behavior, and there are very strong links between the two (exaggerated negative cognitions *probably* lead to emotional disorders). If so, why separate them?

The reasons for our approach are largely to do with scope of practice and the various available interventions for emotional disorders: we believe that, for example, most rehabilitation professionals are well-positioned to address maladaptive cognitions and we've described examples of how in Chapter 10. These include thoughts and understandings, perception, and memory. Yet disorders of emotion or mood, including depression, anxiety, post-traumatic stress, phobia, other impulse control problems, or any of the host of diagnosable psychopathologies described in the *Diagnostic and Statistical Manual of Mental Disorders,* 5th edition (DSM-5) (American Psychiatric Association, 2013), are largely the domain of dedicated mental health professionals. While these things appear to be important drivers of the pain experience for many people, and we sincerely believe that *any* primary care provider should be able to screen for them, the approach to intervention should be different than it is for maladaptive cognitions. In this way we will keep the distinction somewhat simple: if there are diagnostic criteria for it in the current DSM-5 or it has an ICD-10 (or ICD-11 as of 2019) code (usually in the F01-F99 code range), then it will be in the emotional drivers domain. If not, it will be in the cognitive drivers domain. To make it even more clear, there are no diagnostic criteria in the DSM-5 for catastrophizing, perceived injustice, or kinesiophobia, so according to the APT framework these remain squarely in the cognitive domain.

Chapter 11

 The separation of cognitive and emotional drivers in the APT radar plot is admittedly uncommon in pain fields, but is routine in psychological scholarship. By *cognitive* drivers we refer to thoughts, perceptions, memories, executive function and ability to reason and make sense of the world. By *emotional* drivers, we are referring to what are most commonly diagnosable mood disorders, such as depression, anxiety, or phobias. While the former may be amenable to interventions like education or cognitive restructuring techniques, the latter should be addressed by mental health professionals.

So, with that hopefully clarified, let's dive into the proposed mechanisms for the emotional drivers domain. First, it is worth noting that we are not referring here to what could be considered 'normal' or 'rational' negative emotions in reaction to pain. There are very few people who *enjoy* pain and the experience itself is defined as an unpleasant emotional experience, so some degree of fear or sadness in response to pain is both expected and rational. Rather this domain relates to what are commonly considered irrational emotional states, though admittedly what is rational or irrational is highly subjective and the subject of considerable critical social reflection. These emotional states can most commonly be diagnosed as a psychiatric disorder, but may not always meet those criteria (i.e. may be subclinical) or may exist but be undiagnosed. It is also worth noting that decades' worth of research has linked emotional disorders with chronic pain in particular, though the direction of the causal relationship is unclear. Depressive disorders, PTSD, generalized anxiety disorder, somatoform disorder (itself a pain problem), obsessive-compulsive disorders, substance use disorder, and most mental health disorders tend to be over-represented amongst populations with chronic pain, and vice versa (chronic pain tends to be over-represented amongst those with mental health disorders). In short, there

appears to be the potential for some kind of mutual maintenance, and indeed that has been shown for some musculoskeletal pain conditions. For example, in 2018 a group of researchers conducted a systematic review of research exploring the directional links between PTSD and post-traumatic pain, and out of seven studies found quite inconclusive findings, making any concrete commentary on causation quite difficult (Ravn et al., 2018). In other words, it is difficult to state with any confidence whether pain *causes* psychopathology or if psychopathology *causes* pain. As with many such things, the answer is likely 'a little bit of both and it depends on the context', meaning clinicians should be ready and able to identify, and act on, these important health drivers.

The mechanisms to (attempt) to explain the connection between pain and emotional disorders are probably going to be in many ways similar to that of cognitions, though perhaps 'supercharged'. The issues of mood driving the numbers circled on forms, mood driving behavior, and mood driving physiology are likely ramped up even further when it isn't just 'normal' transient negative mood but is rather considered in the context of a full blown, usually irrational, always involuntary, mood disorder.

Fortunately, there is more research to draw on here than there is for maladaptive cognitions, likely because pathological mood disorders have more concrete diagnostic criteria and are more recognizable as public health problems. As mentioned, the *causal* attributions are difficult, but there appear to be at least many shared mechanisms between emotional disorders and chronic pain. For example, genetics research into both conditions has often found that the characteristics of key genes such as *catechol-O-methyltransferase* (COMT) and the 5HT1a (serotonin precursor) receptor have some ability to predict both depression (Taylor et al., 2017) and chronic pain (Fernández-de-las-Peñas et al., 2019; Lee et al., 2018), though the effect appears stronger for the former than the latter. Functional MRI (fMRI) studies have also revealed consistent changes in function and structure of brain regions such as the insular and anterior cingulate cortices that can be seen in both depression (O'Connor & Agius, 2015; Helm et al., 2018) and chronic pain (Wand et al., 2011). The concentrations of some stress markers in the blood or cerebrospinal fluid, such as serotonin and norepinephrine, also appear to be associated with both depression (Brown & Linnoila, 1990) and the response to pain (Martikainen et al., 2018) (perhaps explaining the beneficial effect of some antidepressant medications on chronic pain). Other shared phenomena between mental health disorders and chronic pain include things like disturbed sleep-wake cycles, dysregulated hypothalamic-pituitary-adrenal (HPA) axis activity, impaired higher-level cognitive functioning, and not surprisingly, widespread and non-specific pain. Dysfunction in key cellular, endocrine, or neural pathways will predispose a patient to both hyperalgesia in response to mechanical stimuli and negative mood, regardless of which one is the chicken, and which one is the egg.

A potentially interesting side note here is that many of these phenomena are *also* seen in people with post-concussive syndrome, leading some in the field to opine that some emotional disorders, some chronic pain, and some cortical trauma are not so much distinct conditions but are better conceptualized as different manifestations of some shared mechanism of brain disturbance. The societal and personal implications of this line of thinking are far-reaching and shouldn't be taken lightly, but the suggestions are at least out there and continue to evolve.

So, the mechanisms to explain the link between pain and psychopathology are likely many, very complex, and in some ways, interactive. It should be expected, for example, that someone with an uncontrolled depressive or anxiety disorder will also likely rate themselves as less able to cope with their pain or perform activities in spite of pain, regardless of the functional capacity of their musculoskeletal system. In many ways, depression is characterized itself as an impaired ability to effectively cope in the face of adversity (real or perceived) and a feeling of lethargy or loss of motivation, so one hypothesis for the overlap between pain-related disability and mental health is that the tools used to measure each are not as distinct as we may think. It should also come as no surprise that people who have, or are vulnerable to, a mental health disorder will also feel less resilient in the face of musculoskeletal trauma, and perhaps irrational perceptions of reduced resilience and optimism underlie much of the connection between these two clinical phenomena.

Special considerations

As we are addressing mental health, there are some important considerations for rehabilitation providers who may be under-educated or may not feel confident in their understanding of these topics. The first is the increased prevalence of chronic pain and/or mental health disorders amongst people who report being the victims of interpersonal violence or abuse in either childhood or adulthood. Many large cohort studies have now revealed, among other things, that adverse childhood experiences appear to be risk factors for many health conditions in adulthood, including both chronic pain and psychopathology (Felitti et al., 1998). A history of intimate partner violence in adulthood (physical, emotional, or sexual abuse) also appears to be more common in these two populations. If the current estimate is that 1 in 3 women and 1 in 8 men in the *general population* will have experienced some kind of interpersonal violence, then the proportion in people with chronic pain can be expected to be even higher than that, with some estimates as high as 50% of females (Balousek et al., 2007). This should have important repercussions for healthcare providers working with people with chronic pain, especially those who use personal touch (e.g. massage, manipulation) during treatment. We will circle back around to this in the interventions section below, but we need to be clear that this may be a potential explanation for a patient reporting increased pain following delivery of your seemingly innocuous manual therapy approach. This is also a good time to remind readers of their ethical and legal requirements around mandatory reporting when abuse or violence is disclosed (especially in children), and to brush up on their regulatory obligations in this regard.

Other issues that need to be addressed when discussing mental health are those of addiction and suicide. Again, the degree to which you can and should address these is entirely dependent on your personal context, including what is normal in your field, your training, what other resources are available, and assuming they are able to make sound judgements, what the patient wants. However, we firmly believe that *recognizing the signs* of addiction (better termed *substance use disorder*) and suicidal ideation or risk are critical skills for primary healthcare providers, especially those working with people with chronic pain. Box 11.1 provides some initial guidance and clarification around these issues, but readers are encouraged to seek other opportunities to learn more about these conditions and how to identify and respond within their own personal care contexts.

Distinguishing features

It is difficult to summarize an entire field of research and practice into a few paragraphs, so readers should note that the information provided here is only a superficial overview and they are encouraged to seek out additional training opportunities.

Distinguishing features of mental health disorders can be highly variable both between and within

---

Box 11.1 Suicidal ideation in chronic pain

When a patient discloses thoughts of self-harm or death, healthcare providers have an obligation to explore this further and respond appropriately. A follow-up question to start with is usually something like 'Can you tell me more about these thoughts?' and allow the patient to speak their mind. The clinician is attempting to ascertain whether these are passive thoughts about death or harm, or whether the patient has: 1) *a plan;* and 2) *the means* to carry it out. If the patient does not volunteer this information, more direct questioning is warranted.

In the case of thoughts but no plan, and if the patient is of the age of majority to make their own healthcare decisions, the clinician should ensure they are aware of mental health and suicide prevention resources that can be accessed, and offer to make a referral on the patient's behalf if desired. Additionally, the clinician, depending on context, may offer to contact a family member, clergy, family doctor, friend, or other relevant person, or encourage the patient to do so themselves. A generally good practice (though not always appropriate, so use your judgement) is to also offer to follow-up with the patient by phone in a day or two, at a specific time, and to indicate that if the patient does not answer the phone after two attempts, emergency services will be notified.

In the case of a plan and the means to carry it out, this renders the patient a harm to themselves or others and, in most jurisdictions, is an emergency situation. The clinician should be prepared to contact emergency services and stay with the patient until EMS arrives.

Please note that these represent general guidelines only. Your personal practice context may differ, including regulatory obligations, mandatory reporting, privacy and confidentiality, etc. We encourage you to review these where they exist such that you are prepared in the event that a patient should disclose suicidal ideation.

conditions. For example, someone with persistent mild depression may present quite differently from someone with a bipolar depressive disorder, who themselves could look very different from day to day depending on whether they happen to be in a state of mania or dysthymia. People with a specific phobia may appear to function very normally under most conditions, except in that one situation in which they are confronted with the target of their (usually irrational) fear. A newly described 'dissociative' subtype of PTSD adds additional challenge; where PTSD is often characterized by hypervigilance and physiological arousal in response to traumatic triggers, those with the dissociative subtype may instead present with completely flat affect, go into a sort of dissociative state, and exhibit no obvious reaction to trauma triggers or cues. In some cases, signs of psychopathology are obvious, in other cases they can be hidden either out of shame or intentional manipulation of those around them (in the case of, say, sociopathy), so clinicians may not even be aware. Where they do manifest themselves, many mental health disorders can be characterized by some combination of emotional lability, irrational thoughts, feelings, or behaviors that seem to be out of proportion to the situation when viewing them from the outside (though may seem quite appropriate to the person). Other conditions may present with a spectrum of symptoms including impaired impulse control, whether those be impulsive behaviors (say in the case of obsessive-compulsive, gambling, or eating disorders) or impulsive thoughts (e.g. substance use disorder or depression).

For clinicians not trained in recognizing psychopathology, there are other clues that may crop up during clinical interactions. If the patient's pain experience is being driven primarily by emotion, then you can expect to have difficulty identifying any clear mechanical, inflammatory, or structural pathology to explain the symptoms. Pain provocation tests are likely to be inconsistent or always positive, even

though the pattern doesn't appear to make biomechanical sense. However, findings for things like range of motion or strength *should* be largely within normal limits given the context of the patient's other defining features (age, sex, body habitus, physical fitness, etc.). Palpation may similarly provide very inconsistent results in that it may be that everything hurts or that nothing hurts at all.

More telling for non-mental health professionals would be any number of the existing self-report screening tools available for most (if not all) psychiatric disorders. Tools exist to screen for depression, anxiety, PTSD, phobias, and other disorders. Many have shown adequate diagnostic accuracy to be useful in routine practice, but again only by those providers who are adequately trained in their use and interpretation. Some of the more recognizable tools here include the Patient Health Questionnaire, which has several different versions for screening depression, anxiety, and other health related problems, of which the PHQ-9 depression screen may enjoy the most empirical support. The Beck Depression and Beck Anxiety Inventories are also recognizable in the field, as is the Hospital Anxiety and Depression Scale, the PTSD Checklist, the Depression, Anxiety and Stress Scale, and several others.

The National Institutes of Health in the United States have their own toolbox for mental health disorders, some of which appear to also be useful as screening tools. If we had to predict the total number of tools that have been historically developed for screening mental health disorders it would be easily into the hundreds (perhaps even into the thousands). Accordingly, we will not list them all here, rather we encourage readers to seek out a couple of such tools that would be relevant for their contexts, ensuring that they have been tested for use in samples of similar age, culture, language, and healthcare context as your own patients. It is of course important to state that you are not required to administer the tool to patients if you don't feel

	Suggested evidence for triangulation: emotional domain	
Test domains	**Findings**	**Shift in likelihood**
Screening tools	Several tools are widely available, intended to screen for psychopathology in adults. These include tools for: depression (PHQ-9, BDI and BDI-II, Zung Depression Rating Scale, Hamilton Depression Rating Scale, Hospital Anxiety and Distress Scale), generalized anxiety disorder (GAD-7, HADS, BAI), PTSD (IES, PCL, PDS), and several tools that are intended to screen for multiple psychopathologies including: the Depression, Anxiety and Stress Scale (DASS), the General Health Questionnaire 28 (GHQ-28), and the full version of the Patient Health Questionnaire. Note that some tools, such as the Beck Depression and Beck Anxiety Indices, the PDS and the GHQ-28 are copyrighted and therefore either require permission or payment to use. Almost all of the psychological screening tools are more sensitive than specific, meaning they are more accurate for saying that psychopathology does NOT exist than they are for saying it does, and that false positives are common. Hence, triangulate.	++
Symptom behavior	Symptom behavior is more likely linked to emotions, where pain will most commonly increase in the presence of heightened depression, or perhaps during periods of sleep disturbance (worse sleep, more pain). Anxiety may also lead to increased pain experience, though it is possible that during an acute anxiety or panic attack, pain sensitivity/intensity is reduced.	+
Palpation	Despite what we are not calling a strong nociceptive component here, don't be surprised to find considerable tenderness to palpation. This type of sign will overlap with the *central nociplastic* domain, in that you may well find diffuse, widespread tenderness to palpation that is not associated with any single tissue	Neutral
Quantitative sensory testing	The results here will best be described as inconclusive, and perhaps inconsistent dependent on the person's emotional state at the time of testing. As with palpation, you may identify widespread non-dermatomal sensory hypersensitivity across testing modalities (mechanical, cold, heat), and people with anxiety or depression disorders also often report sensitivity to environmental stimuli like odor, light, and ambient temperature. Beyond 'inconsistent', QST is unlikely to shed much light on a strong emotional driver.	Neutral
Sensorimotor testing	Pain with a strong emotional driver is unlikely to present with clear signs of sensorimotor dysintegration, or when they do appear, they are likely to again be inconsistent at best. This shouldn't be taken to mean that the person is somehow faking their performance on the test, rather, remember that all of these tests, also including palpation, QST, and mechanical testing, rely on accurate patient report as part of the interpretation of the results. As such these are best considered psychophysical tests, meaning that labile emotions or inaccurate perceptions of the world may lead to findings that are difficult to interpret.	Neutral

Suggested evidence for triangulation: emotional domain *continued*

Test domains	Findings	Shift in likelihood
Mechanical testing	Pain with a strong emotional driver will not follow any clear 'mechanical' or 'inflammatory' (nociceptive) patterns. Those with irrational fear of movement (a true 'phobia') or related anxiety are likely to report pain prior to its actual onset, not out of intentional malingering but out of a genuine belief (though perhaps inaccurate) that pushing farther will result in pain they are unable to manage. Expect reduced range and early reports of pain on many of your clinical mechanical tests, though these are unlikely related to any specific mechanical dysfunction. As such, the 'positive' test in this domain is non-mechanical, inconsistent results of mechanical testing, overlapping considerably with the *cognitive* domain.	+
Cognitions	Ask 10 different psychological researchers and you'll likely get 10 different answers on this one, but for our purposes we're going to consider exaggerated negative or maladaptive cognitions both a precursor to frank psychopathology and a symptom thereof. So, it will be awfully strange to see a patient who has a depressive or anxiety disorder who does *not* also score higher than average on your pain cognitions tools, like the Pain Catastrophizing Scale or Tampa Scale for Kinesiophobia. This probably speaks to a slight issue with measurement theory and design, but we'll not go too far down that rabbit hole here. For our purposes let's assume that cognitive tools will be highly sensitive but not very specific for mood-based psychopathology.	+
Emotions	By definition this is the most telling domain, though the self-report screening tools should also be used to triangulate your clinical impression. For those who are unfamiliar with the field of psychology, there are some important considerations here. First of all, just because someone has depression doesn't mean they're always crying or suicidal any more than someone with an anxiety disorder is always shaking and panicking. There are very many people in this world who have, or could meet the criteria for, some kind of psychopathology yet are functioning perfectly well in daily life. In fact, some scholars have argued that many historical figures in high-ranking positions of power also very likely suffer or suffered from some kind of mood, impulse, or personality disorder. Signs and symptoms here are probably going to be more subtle than most, and you may or may not ever pick them up. However, in the case that a patient presents with a *purely* emotional driver for their pain experience, that would suggest higher dysfunction than most people. These people may present as emotionally labile either day-to-day or even moment-to-moment. Some may appear to interpret every daily event in the worst possible light, or express very little in the way of hope or optimism. A person with PTSD may react in odd, unexpected, or occasionally (and very rarely) violent ways in reaction to seemingly benign comments or questions. True diagnosis requires a trained mental health professional, however, pain that appears to have no clear connection with movement or activity but seems to vary along with emotions would be a key sign here.	+++

—*continued*—

Test domains	Findings	Shift in likelihood
	Suggested evidence for triangulation: emotional domain *continued*	
Socioenvironmental	Mental health disorders can affect people from all walks of life, so any comments made here are at best broad generalizations rather than strict rules or guidelines. Epidemiological evidence consistently reveals that those with emotional disorders also tend to come from lower socioeconomic backgrounds, have lower educational attainment, and have less effective social support networks, though these are averages rather than rules or facts. Evidence from large prospective cohort studies like the *Adverse Childhood Experiences* (ACE) study have also shown a link between early life adversity (or even prenatal maternal stress) and psychopathology in adult life. While causality is always hard to prove, there is strong evidence that early life adversity precedes adult psychopathology, and that psychopathology in adulthood also precedes problems with work, finances, and interpersonal connections. And, perhaps not surprisingly, almost all of these have consistent associations with pain intensity.	+
Pathology	One of the hallmarks of this domain, like the cognitive domain, will be the absence of clear structural pathology to explain the symptoms. Where biological markers are identifiable in psychopathology they tend to be in the form of blood- or saliva-based markers of stress system dysregulation or non-routine static or dynamic ('functional') brain imaging studies. Even these however are not diagnostic as many health conditions can masquerade with the same biological profiles as psychopathology, and vice versa. While biological testing may lend some support to the presence of psychopathology when present along with other signs and symptoms, it is not currently, as of this writing, recommended as a diagnostic or screening approach. The most useful evidence for triangulation in this domain then would be an absence of clear structural pathology to explain the pain-related symptoms.	+

comfortable doing so, and in fact if you do feel uncomfortable or not adequately trained, we'd encourage you to avoid using such scales until you have received more training. Even becoming familiar with the items on the form and what the criteria are for a 'positive' screen is a good first step as doing so will help you to identify those potentially concerning statements that patients can and will make, cueing you to the possible existence of an undiagnosed mental health disorder.

Prognostic Value

In Chapter 10 we stated that cognitive factors were amongst the most common predictors of outcome in both acute and chronic pain states, so it should come

as no surprise that emotional factors, themselves perhaps most easily considered the 'outcomes' of cognitions, also enjoy the same predictive value. Of those, depression is likely the single most common predictor of pain and related disability that persist after acute trauma or that do not respond well to intervention (Walton et al., 2013; Linton, 2000). This includes both fairly simple yes/no (present/absent) type factors for depression, as well as scores on scales of depression magnitude such as the PHQ-9, BDI, or HADS.

In conditions that can be traced back to trauma as their genesis, post-traumatic stress symptoms are also common prognostic factors for pain and recovery (Pedler & Sterling, 2013; McLean et al., 2005).

It should be noted that PTSD as a psychiatric diagnosis cannot, according to DSM-5 criteria, be made until the symptoms of hyperarousal, intrusion, and avoidance have been present for at least one month. Prior to that, a separate diagnosis, called *Acute Stress Disorder*, *can* be made, though it is made more rarely. Self-report screening tools are available for identifying the condition, including the Acute Stress Disorder Scale (ASDS) (Bryant et al., 2000) and the Stanford Acute Stress Reaction Questionnaire (ASRQ) (Cardeña et al., 2000). Often considered a precursor to (or at least a risk factor for) PTSD, the symptoms are largely similar between the two, with ASDS being diagnosable in the shorter term after a traumatic event. When present, both are likely predictive of poor recovery.

Generalized anxiety disorder (GAD) is another that has shown some evidence of predictive value, though not as strong as other psychopathologies. If anxieties are irrational fears of something terrible happening, then it stands to reason that those with uncontrolled anxiety disorders are also at risk of reporting other terrible things such as ongoing pain and disability, though the mechanism for such shouldn't be assumed to be due to irrational thought *per se*. It is possible that exaggerated anxiety, often accompanied by a sort of persistent 'fight, flight or freeze' state, may lead to avoidance of triggering contexts (such as social spaces or exercise) that could lead to a state of disuse, deconditioning, and atrophy. Similarly, the maintained anxiety may also lead to an over-active (but under-effective) hypothalamic-pituitary-adrenal axis, or sympathetic-adrenal-medullary axis, that pump cortisol or adrenaline (respectively) into the system. Phobias, a subtype of anxiety disorders characterized by irrational fear of usually something fairly specific (e.g. heights, spiders, flying, injury) may also be related to poor functional outcomes and reports of pain especially in the presence of the feared stimulus or context. These have not been traditionally studied in pain conditions, with the arguable exception of kinesiophobia (irrational fear of movement/(re)injury), though this is not in fact a diagnosable psychopathology.

Personality disorders, including borderline personality disorder, narcissistic, avoidant, dependent, obsessive-compulsive, and schizoid, enjoyed some research attention in the 1980s, 90s and early 2000s, though have not since been a big focus of pain research. This is partly because personality inventories are usually very long and require considerable training to administer and interpret properly, and partly because most clinicians don't really know how intervention should be different or modified in the presence of a positive finding (so a large burden for comparatively little value). When they were explored, mostly in low back pain and somewhat in neck pain, not surprisingly those who showed more 'disordered' personality types were also the ones who tended to report lower treatment effectiveness (Love & Peck, 1987), but there is so much overlap across these psychological domains that it is hard to find the chicken and the egg in this area of study.

On balance, as per cognitive factors, the more someone rates higher on scales of psychopathology (including emotional and personality disorders), the more likely that person is also going to rate higher on scales of pain and functional interference concurrently and longitudinally. Mechanisms are yet to be fully sorted out, though there are several potential hypotheses from disordered thinking patterns and perceptual deficits through psychoneuroendocrine pathways that may at least partly explain the associations between current psychopathology and future pain.

Intervention strategies

In the presence of verifiable psychopathology, or even suspected psychopathology, the intervention for that condition as a primary driver of a patient's pain experience should be the fairly exclusive domain of mental health professionals. Intervention strategies most commonly take the form of one-on-one talk-based therapies ('counseling'), behavior monitoring, awareness, thought monitoring and control approaches (cognitive-behavioral therapy), mindfulness or other centering and presence techniques, pharmaceuticals, group classes, or support groups. Some other more intensive approaches include inpatient or day programs, transcranial or electroconvulsive stimulation, or even implantable electrodes for deep brain stimulation in extreme cases. Talk-based therapies and counseling with or without pharmaceuticals are common first-line therapies, and new evidence from multi- or interdisciplinary treatment settings are finding that these interventions combined with physical interventions like exercise, sleep hygiene, stress inoculation with exercise, or behavior modification can be more effective when delivered as part of a comprehensive treatment plan than when each are delivered in isolation. Clinicians are encouraged to educate themselves about mental health disorders and the resources available in their local and virtual (online or tele-medicine/ rehabilitation services) communities, and to engage with other disciplinary practitioners to explore more holistic intervention strategies for patients in pain where a strong emotional component is believed to be the primary driver.

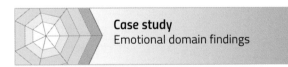

Case study
Emotional domain findings

Returning to our case of Sean, it is time to conduct an appropriate (and appropriately sensitive) exploration of possible emotional or mood disorders. As you broach the subject, Sean indicates that he does have a diagnosis of depression and has been on 50mg of sertraline (an SSRI) for several years. Through the medication and occasional visits with a counselor he indicates that the depression is well-controlled, though admits that the past few days have been 'very hard' since the event. Knowing that he already has been diagnosed, we may not need to conduct much further exploration of this domain. The harder question however is the degree to which we believe the depression may be *contributing to* his pain experience, and thus, make it a reasonable target for intervention (if appropriate). This can be a difficult call to make at the time, and sometimes the only way to know if a psychological intervention will also reduce pain, is to try it. But for the sake of our case, let's assume that if his depression has been well-controlled for a couple of years, then presumably he should currently score *under* threshold on a validated depression screen. If he scores over threshold, and in light of his comments that he has found himself struggling to manage his emotions since the event, we would be justified in considering the emotional domain a relatively stronger driver of his pain experience.

Turning to the literature, we identify the well-validated Patient Health Questionnaire-9 item version, which is a self-report tool with questions taken almost verbatim from the current diagnostic criteria for major depressive disorder (scoring algorithms can be found fairly easily online, though be aware that it's not particularly straightforward). In this case, Sean scores positive for major depressive disorder, a result about which he is not surprised. After a short conversation explaining the potential for mutual maintenance between uncontrolled depression and pain (but not adding to the shame often experienced by those with a mental health disorder), Sean agrees to reconnect with his counselor and explore with his doctor the possibility of a short course of an increased dose of sertraline or a different class of drug altogether to try to address his emotional status.

In light of this information, in relative terms, we're going to reduce the relative contributions from the maladaptive cognitions *a little* and make the emotional driver the higher priority at this time (Fig. 11.1).

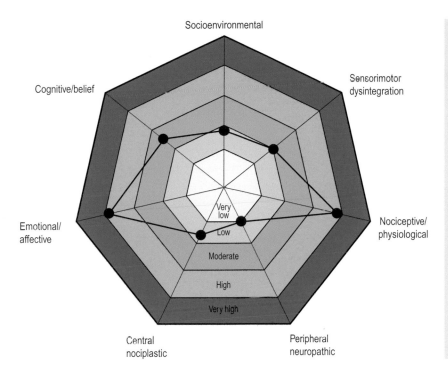

Figure 11.1
Sean's radar plot continues to take shape. Based on the emotional domain findings, this driver has been moved to 'high' probability, and the cognitive domain driver has been moved down to 'moderate' from the previous 'high' probability.

References

American Psychiatric Association, 2013. Diagnostic and statistical manual of mental disorders (5th ed.). American Psychiatric Association; Washington, DC.

Balousek, S., Plane, M. B., Fleming, M., 2007. Prevalence of interpersonal abuse in primary care patients prescribed opioids for chronic pain. *Journal of General Internal Medicine* 22 (9):1268–73.

Brown, G. L., Linnoila, M. I., 1990. CSF serotonin metabolite (5-HIAA) studies in depression, impulsivity, and violence. *The Journal of Clinical Psychiatry* 51 (Suppl):31-41; discussion 42–3.

Bryant, R. A., Moulds, M. L., Guthrie, R. M., 2000. Acute Stress Disorder Scale: a self-report measure of acute stress disorder. *Psychological Assessment* 12 (1):61–8.

Cardeña, E., Koopman, C., Classen, C., et al., 2000. Psychometric properties of the Stanford Acute Stress Reaction Questionnaire (SASRQ): a valid and reliable measure of acute stress. *Journal of Traumatic Stress* 13 (4):719–34.

Felitti, V. J., Anda, R. F., Nordenberg, D., et al., 1998. Relationship of childhood abuse and household dysfunction to many of the leading causes of death in adults. The Adverse Childhood Experiences (ACE) Study. *American Journal of Preventive Medicine* 14 (4):245–58.

Fernández-de-las-Peñas, C., Ambite-Quesada, S., Palacios-Ceña, M., et al., 2019. Catechol-O-Methyltransferase (COMT) rs4680 Val158Met polymorphism is associated with widespread pressure pain sensitivity and depression in women with chronic, but not episodic, tension-type headache. *The Clinical Journal of Pain* 35 (4):345–52.

Helm, K., Viol, K., Weiger, T. M., et al., 2018. Neuronal connectivity in major depressive disorder: a systematic review. *Neuropsychiatric Disease and Treatment* 17 (14):2715–37. Available at: https://www.dovepress.com/neuronal-connectivity-in-major-depressive-disorder-a-systematic-review-peer-reviewed-article-NDT.

Lee, C., Liptan, G., Kantorovich, S., et al., 2018. Association of Catechol-O-methyltransferase single nucleotide polymorphisms, ethnicity, and sex in a large cohort of fibromyalgia patients. *BMC Rheumatology* 2 (1):38.

Linton, S. J., 2000. A review of psychological risk factors in back and neck pain. *Spine*, 25(9):1148–56.

Love, A. W., Peck, C. L., 1987. The MMPI and psychological factors in chronic low back pain: a review. *Pain* 28 (1):1–12.

Martikainen, I. K., Hagelberg, N., Jääskeläinen, S. K. et al., 2018. Dopaminergic and serotonergic mechanisms in the modulation of pain: In vivo studies in human brain. *European Journal of Pharmacology* 834:337–45.

McLean, S. A., Clauw, D. J., Abelson, J. L.,et al., 2005. The development of persistent pain and psychological morbidity after motor vehicle collision: integrating the potential role of stress response systems into a biopsychosocial model. *Psychosomatic Medicine* 67 (5):783–90.

O'Connor, S., Agius, M., 2015. A systematic review of structural and functional MRI differences between psychotic and nonpsychotic depression. *Psychiatria Danubina* 27 (Suppl 1):S235-9.

Pedler, A., Sterling, M., 2013. Patients with chronic whiplash can be subgrouped on the basis of symptoms of sensory hypersensitivity and posttraumatic stress. *Pain* 154 (9):1640–8.

Ravn, S. L., Hartvigsen, J., Hansen, M., et al., 2018. Do post-traumatic pain and post-traumatic stress symptomatology mutually maintain each other? A systematic review of cross-lagged studies. *Pain* 159 (11):2159–69.

Taylor, M. K., Beckerley, S. E., Henniger, N. E., et al., 2017. A genetic risk factor for major depression and suicidal ideation is mitigated by physical activity. *Psychiatry Research* 249:304–6.

Walton, D. M., Macdermid, J. C., Giorgianni, A. A., et al., 2013. Risk factors for persistent problems following acute whiplash injury: update of a systematic review and meta-analysis. *The Journal of Orthopaedic and Sports Physical Therapy* 43 (2):31–43.

Wand, B. M., Parkitny, L., O'Connell, N. E., et al., 2011. Cortical changes in chronic low back pain: current state of the art and implications for clinical practice. *Manual Therapy* 16 (1):15–20.

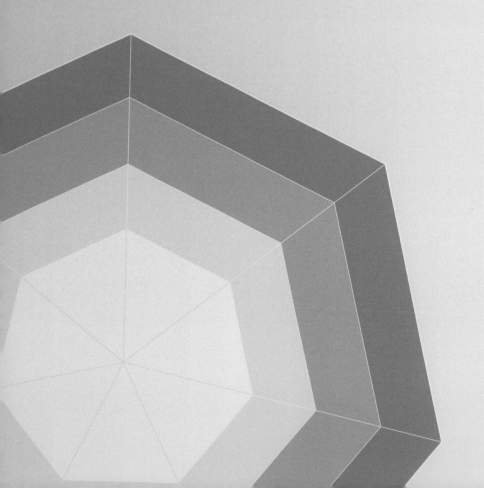

12

The Socioenvironmental Domain

Proposed mechanisms

This domain could easily get so large as to be somewhat overwhelming. We are talking about what we believe to be the ENTIRETY of the social and environmental contexts within which health, pain, illness, and disability occur, and how they are interpreted. In fact, many historic scholars have highlighted how disability itself is a social construct, insofar as people are only considered 'disabled' when some aspect of their being, agency, or ability does not conform to social constructions of 'normal'. There are powerful influences on our current conceptualizations of and acceptance for terms like normal and disabled, including medical, governmental, economic, and educational powers. The very label of 'disabled' carries tremendous gravitas and impact for the person being labelled, affecting their access to and types of care provided, opportunities for productive occupation, and influences on interpersonal dynamics. A full social discourse on the concepts of disability is well beyond what can be logically included in the pages of this book, though the academic literature is rich with disability scholars to which interested readers are directed. We are going to necessarily take a narrowed view of the issue by focusing more on common illustrative examples of how social and environmental pressures can influence the experience of pain and disability, while being fully transparent that any such undertaking is superficial in this context.

The first thing that needs to be stated here is that a rating or description of one's pain is itself a pain behavior. That is, the decision of whether you answer '4' or '7' to the request for a rating between 0 and 10 is influenced by far more factors than the 'real' severity of the pain, assuming there is one single real reality of your pain and that you're able to access it. Earlier sections have addressed things like genetic sensitivity or emotional state as influencing what number on the 0-10 scale you choose. Arguably one of, if not the largest, influence is the interpersonal context in which the question is being asked. A pain rating is a transaction between you and your patient, and like any social transaction, will be influenced by social biases

(perceived or real) including how the patient wants to be perceived. These could include how they feel about you as a person or as a professional, how they think you'll react to different numbers, how strong they want to appear or how vulnerable, what they believe your agenda may be, what they think of your profession on the whole, and how they think your decisions around treatment will be affected by the number they provide. This is simply a truism of any social encounter, and we can say with confidence the exact same things influence your response if and when another healthcare provider was to ask *you* about *your* pain or other symptoms.

 We have consistently found that the mean numeric rating of pain intensity across populations and conditions is *most commonly* between 4 and 6 out of 10, with a standard deviation between 1.5 and 2.5. Go ahead and look it up now if you like: find an RCT studying an intervention for a sample of people in pain, check the baseline pain scores displayed in the study's table, and see if we're right. Assuming that's the case, it begs the question of why? Why is the average pain score that patients give so commonly in the middle of the scale? Is it because the single-item 0-10 Numeric Rating Scale is one of the most psychometrically sound tools ever created? Probably not. Our belief is that this is a phenomenon of social interactivity. That is, patients are likely having internal dialogues like: 'If I rate too high this person may not believe me, but if I rate too low they may not treat me', or 'If I start in the middle, then I'll have some room to move either direction depending on what they offer me', or even 'What number does this person need to hear in order to give me the treatment I need?' In this way, we and others recognize a pain intensity score as a transaction between patient and provider that is driven at least as much by social factors as by any biological factors.

It has been shown that pain ratings can be influenced by the sex of the patient and provider, the perceived attractiveness of the provider (independent of sex), the perceived competence of the provider, the patient's perceptions of things like empathy, tone of voice, and connection, as well as the degree to which they feel their complaints have been heard and validated. To be clear this is not an exact or even an objective science. Pain ratings are by nature subjective, just as pain itself is subjective, meaning that ratings and other behaviors (limping, grimacing, vocalizing, etc.) are all going to be influenced by the nature of your connection with the patient. There is no such thing as a true unbiased pain rating – we might as well just accept that now.

Below we will describe just a few of the various social or contextual influences that have been shown to have an effect on things like pain persistence or pain severity. The illustrative examples we will choose to explore here include gender-based norms and roles, ethnocultural influences (where those have been explored objectively enough to be discussed critically), education, socioeconomic status, medicolegal context, and pre-trauma adversity. We are therefore *not* discussing things such as diet, climate, religion and spirituality, industry and job opportunities, governmental policies and practices, or structural barriers (e.g. stairs, hills, sidewalks, etc.) among many others. We will also focus on how the socioenvironmental influences we discuss are likely to affect the experience or reporting of the patient's *pain* specifically, intentionally leaving reported pain-related disability for other forums.

Gender

Starting with gender, we first need to ensure the terminology here is clear. We are using the definition of gender as described by the World Health Organization: *the socially constructed characteristics of women and men – such as norms, roles and relationships of and between groups of women and men.* This differs from sex in that the term 'sex' most commonly refers to the biological differences between males and females including chromosomes, hormones, and reproductive organs, while gender refers more to the social and cultural 'norms' traditionally associated with the

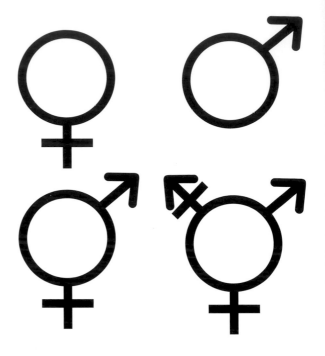

sexes, such as masculinity and femininity. As we have already touched on this in Chapter 4, we can be fairly brief as there is consistent evidence to support a difference in pain sensitivity, perception or expression, between men and women. Less clear is whether this difference can be explained by biological differences between the sexes such as neural processing, endocrine (hormonal) influences, or differences in nociceptor-innervated tissue proportion and distribution, or can be better explained by social mechanisms, such as willingness to report pain, feel and express empathy, or interpersonal connectedness. The current state of evidence precludes us from making any definitive statements on this matter, and in reality, the truth is probably some combination of both sex and gender and the interactions between them. For the purposes of this chapter and in recognizing that we are writing from a largely Eurocentric or 'Western' cultural perspective, we will borrow from common parlance and state that traditionally feminine gender traits *tend* towards greater propensity to express pain and seek support from others, while traditionally masculine traits *tend* towards suppression of pain and stoicism, which may at least partly explain the differences. This is a dramatic oversimplification of a very complex and diverse field of study, and not necessarily views that we hold ourselves, but will do for now to ground our further discussion.

When exploring sex or gender as a driver of a pain experience, astute clinicians are more likely to identify other areas that may be amenable to intervention and that have been traditionally described as 'genderized'. These could include the traditional tendency for females to bear more of the work of child-rearing and domestic duties, that, when combined with the rising rate of females working outside of the home, may point to a potential mechanism driving pain. In this theory, the driver is less about feminine propensities towards connectedness, expression, and social support; rather pain is driven by reduced 'down time' for females with therefore greater allostatic[1] load on tissues that is not conducive to rest and recovery.

In the move towards 'personalized medicine' we've yet to reach a level of knowledge that could help clinicians make sex- or gender-based decisions about pain treatment, but more on that in the following sections. As an interesting side-note here, it is worth mentioning that while females tend to be over-represented in most chronic pain conditions, the majority of pain research (especially animal research) has primarily been performed on males. Even in human research, women were historically excluded from studies due to a pervasive belief at the time (by the largely male world of researchers) that hormonal fluctuations would add undesirable 'noise' to their otherwise well-constructed studies. This meant that, rather than attempting to explore and understand these influences, there were instead simply ignored. While this trend has improved dramatically over the past two decades,

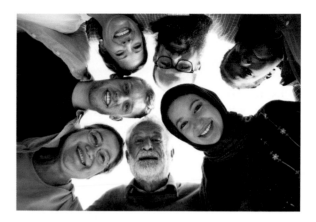

some notable exclusions persist to this day, such as the common practice of excluding pregnant women. Once again, this means we know very little about how treatment decisions ought to be made when pregnant women develop pain. Collectively, there's an increasingly recognized problem pain research regarding sex and gender, which is to say we know very little about how, if at all, treatments should differ between males and females.

Ethnocultural background

There have been some attempts to explore ethnocultural influences on pain reports, though most (perhaps all) are still in the correlation rather than causation stage, leaving any such discussion vulnerable to alternative explanations and an acknowledged risk of harmful stigma that we will try to avoid. Where they have been explored, there is somewhat consistent evidence that an association or difference exists in pain reporting between people of European Caucasian descent (often referred to as non-Hispanic white), those from African backgrounds (often referred to as black), and those from East Asian background (e.g. China, Japan, Korea). For example, Fuentes and colleagues (Fuentes et al., 2007) conducted a series

---

[1] Chronic exposure to elevated or fluctuating endocrine or neural responses resulting from chronic or repeated challenges that the individual experiences as stressful. It is the 'wear and tear' on the body.

of advanced modeling analyses on a sample of over 2,000 older white and black adults and found that the black adults tended to rate higher pain interference, but the relationship was far from obviously causal, especially when they also found that pain interference was influenced by socioeconomic status. Ahn and colleagues (Ahn et al., 2017) compared 50 Asian Americans to 50 age- and sex-matched non-Hispanic whites, all with knee osteoarthritis, to find that the Asian group reported higher pain intensity and were more pain sensitive in response to standardized quantitative sensory tests. There are several other such findings and we need not explore them all to make the point that prior evidence has, fairly consistently identified what are described as racial or ethnic differences in pain severity or sensitivity.

While biological differences, such as genetics, *could* explain variability in pain processing, our collective understanding of the precise underlying mechanisms is still very much in its infancy. It is however, plausible that other social or cultural influences are contributing to these differences. One such example could be differences in traditional dietary habits across cultures. The diversity of the gut microbiome (the type and variety of bacteria in your gut) is starting to show associations with pain sensitivity, and may explain some cultural differences as a result of prevailing dietary habits. Differences in daily activity, environmental exposures (e.g. hours of sunlight, temperature fluctuations, exposure to environmental disasters), and lifetime access to healthcare (including thousands of other factors) between people living in different global regions could all explain at least some component of these reported differences.

One could also raise the argument that the tools used for measuring pain, themselves tremendously vulnerable to bias and inaccuracy, are not adequately comparable across languages (despite several having undergone rigorous language translations) and

it may be that it's the difference in measurement tool properties that explains the differences between cultures. As a point of clarity, the majority of pain-related measurement tools have been designed and evaluated in populations that are dominated by non-Hispanic white participants with largely Eurocentric or North American values. So in other words, perhaps it's not the participants in the study, it's the tool being used that explains these differences.

If gender-based pain decisions are hard to come by given the current state of knowledge, ethnocultural-based decisions are even more elusive.

Educational attainment

As we continue what are primarily theoretical discussions in these domains, you will likely start to recognize potential juncture points where one socio-environmental domain may be influencing, or confounding, another. Educational attainment is no doubt one of those. There is considerable empirical evidence to indicate an inverse association between years of education and likelihood of a chronic pain problem (people who have more education are less likely to develop chronic pain). For example, one of our own meta-analyses in whiplash found that those with no post-secondary education were more likely to describe persistent pain and related symptoms 12 months following the trauma. More recent work in our labs is indicating that educational attainment interacts in interesting ways with other predictors of recovery, such as post-traumatic distress, which essentially means the risk posed by PTSD is magnified in those without a post-secondary education. But, caution is required when interpreting such findings. As with any of the phenomena in this section, correlation should not be conflated with causation. While people with lower education attainment may be more likely to describe chronic pain and disability than those with a higher education, the critical question is why? Are people with less education more likely to misinterpret 'normal' sensations as harmful or painful? Are they less able to understand physiological processes or anatomy, and therefore more prone to catastrophic beliefs about the potential impact of pain? Are there fewer alternative job opportunities available to those with less education, meaning they are more likely to be impacted by pain and more likely to stay on wage indemnity benefits longer than those who could more easily find other options? Is there an influence of comprehension and interpretation of common pain and disability measurement tools that leads those with lower education to circle numbers on the form to indicate greater severity? Clearly, the story is 'as clear as mud'.

In some ways, all such questions around why people with lower education attainment may be more likely to have chronic pain and disability likely have an element of truth. Yet they all seem overly simplistic as well. An additional interesting question could be: '*Why* did that person not attend a post-secondary educational institution?' Now the potential mechanisms at play towards explaining the influence of education on pain expands considerably. Educational attainment itself is probably best considered as a proxy for some other mechanisms, such as geography, socioeconomic status, cultural norms regarding education of women or girls, teen pregnancy rates, among many others. We can start to see where the touch points exist between several socioenvironmental domains, and the tremendous complexity (and perhaps foolishness) of trying to dissect them one-by-one. Even now in 2019 the proportions of white to black students in post-secondary education in North America is highly unbalanced: could this be the mechanism for the ethnocultural differences described above? Or vice versa? Where is the chicken and where is the egg in any of these relationships? People who live in a city that does not have a post-secondary institution are less likely to attend college or university than are those who live

near such an institution. Perhaps not coincidentally, cities with post-secondary institutions are also more likely to have secondary or tertiary-level healthcare facilities. Working backwards, the explanation may well be that those people who report greater pain severity have also had less access to effective pain management, as they live in a city with neither specialist care nor easy access to post-secondary education, and there's your connection. Clearly, we could hypothesize in circles on the potential mechanisms at play here, and there are yet far more questions than answers.

Socioeconomic status

Social ethnographers and epidemiologists have provided considerable evidence that the *best* predictor of successful outcomes following surgery are not sex, BMI, age, or even duration of pre-surgical pain, but zip/postal code. So powerful has socioeconomic status as a determinant of many health conditions become that National Institutes of Health Director Dr. Francis Collins has endorsed the notion of 'ZNA' to explain health; that is, 'zip code DNA'. And while it would be another over-simplification to state that the only difference between zip codes is the median income of its residents, this is no doubt a strong discriminator. Moreover, if we were to dig deeper, perhaps it has less to do with 'ZNA', but rather what street you live on, in that prosperous neighborhoods have social resources that others do not. This includes, but is not limited to, access to fresh and nutritious foods, parks and playgrounds, cleaner air, high-quality schools, civil services, security, neighborhood connectedness, and many others.

Again, the mechanisms will be tremendously complex and we'll do justice to none of them by trying to tease them all apart here. One interesting finding however is that socioeconomic status (SES) appears to predict health status (including pain severity and recovery) regardless of the healthcare funding model. In other words, this is not a phenomenon isolated to

Chapter 12

private healthcare settings: those in fully socialized healthcare environments like Canada still find very similar phenomena. So, the issue cannot be simply reduced to the differences in ability to pay for healthcare services rendered. A reasonable hypothesis is that those who live on the margins of financial stability are more vulnerable to considerable distress by even a temporary loss of income-earning potential, and so we could return to prior discussions around the relationship between distress and pain as a potential mechanism here. Another very germane observation is that lower SES is a risk factor for several chronic health conditions, not just pain, so the generally higher ratings of pain severity or greater risk of chronic pain may simply be indicators of the apparent vulnerability to any number of chronic health conditions. For example, we also identify the existence of comorbid health conditions such as diabetes, depression, and obesity (to name very few) predicting pain severity and recovery. As such, it is once again possible that low SES is a proxy variable in research studies that is actually describing people in terms of comorbidities, other life stressors, and health literacy rather than a smaller bank balance.

Medicolegal context

As Dr. Nortin M. Hadler observed in 1996: "*You cannot get well if you have to constantly prove you are ill*" (Hadler, 1996). Pain, especially from a traumatic onset (e.g. work-related injury, abuse, assault, medical malpractice cases, motor vehicle collision), tends to occur in highly litigious environments. Whether the perceived result of a work-related injury, a motor vehicle collision, or someone else's negligence, many people in pain will also be involved in some form of legal or insurance proceeding that appears to be associated with pain severity. It almost goes without saying by now that the mechanisms to explain the association are complex. But, it feels particularly important to explore this in slightly greater detail here.

Our experience in speaking with audiences around the world has revealed that healthcare providers carry a healthy dose of skepticism towards people in pain who also have an active legal or insurance case. And it only makes sense of course, any time there is potential for financial loss or gain, the person at the center of it all cannot be unbiased. We're not sure why anyone would expect they could be. Indeed, we ourselves probably embellish our stories of illness slightly when we go to see our own doctors about an unknown condition, even when we have no financial stake in it personally. Clearly those who do have financial security to lose or gain should be expected to do what needs to be done to ensure their story is heard. It would be naïve to think otherwise, if for no other reason than they can rest assured the team on the opposing side will be embellishing every bit as strongly to disprove the reported and documented pain exists. These may be the mechanisms behind findings reported from countries such as Lithuania, Turkey, Holland, and Greece, that suggest the phenomenon of chronic whiplash-associated disorder (WAD) does not exist in those countries *because* there exists neither the mechanisms nor expectations of any kind of compensation following a car crash. These studies are very often submitted as evidence to support calls to reduce, or even eliminate, funding for healthcare following such traumas, using arguments such as: "*On the basis of [data from Lithuania, Germany and Greece] one could really question the validity of any claim of chronic injury in WAD Grade 1 or 2*" (Ferrari et al., 1999, pg. 326). On a more personal note, we are reminded of an invited speaking engagement we provided a couple of years back on WAD, after which a member of the audience, an aged medical practitioner with considerable experience conducting 'independent medical evaluations' for insurance companies, stood and opined: "*I'll tell you what will cure these people with whiplash – a pile of $100 bills*", to which a few of his colleagues yelped: "*Hear, hear!*" It would be dangerous to suggest these sentiments are wrong in all cases as there no doubt exists the odd rogue patient who is trying to feign their symptoms for financial gain. But, safe to say, there's a lot of work needed before the 'belief-gaps' can be narrowed.

While the legal and insurance systems are intended to support those who have been unfairly victimized by negligence or injustice, the reality is that going through that experience is tremendously stressful. When combined with the distress of being in pain in the first place, it should come as little surprise that those engaged in such processes rate their pain and disability as more severe. Yet to say that the mechanism is purely due to 'secondary gain', with the over-arching desire to score a nice payout, seems simplistic and unfair in the vast majority of cases. And, accruing evidence supports some mechanism beyond intentional exaggeration or 'malingering' that is driving the pain experience. For example, Australian researchers followed a sample of 155 people from within weeks of a car crash to 12 months later and modeled the trajectories within their recovery data. They found that in those that were in the least impaired (least severe) recovery trajectory, initiating a new medicolegal claim did in fact coincide with a 'bump-up' in their pain and disability severity ratings. Yet those who were in the most impaired (most severe) trajectory showed no change in pain or disability with the initiation of a claim. In other words, initiating a claim seems to really only have an observable impact in those who appeared to be on an otherwise good path, but if the person was on track towards chronic pain from the early acute phase, the claim had no effect on self-reported pain and disability. The Canadian researcher Dr. Natalie Spearing and her colleagues, have conducted rigorous syntheses of the research in this area and, after having parsed, appraised, and synthesized it, have arrived at a largely similar position to ours – that being involved in an active litigation case does appear to be associated with higher ratings of pain and disability, but

they are unable to find any indication that this association is explained by intentional exaggeration for financial gain (Spearing, et al., 2012a; Spearing et al., 2012b; Spearing & Connelly, 2011).

This does beg the question: if intentional exaggeration is *not* a primary driver in the majority of patients with an active claim, what is? It is important to remember that the direction of causation is unclear in most work from the field. Is it the case that people who get involved in medicolegal action suddenly rate their pain higher, or is it that those who have more severe pain are more likely to initiate medicolegal action? This question has yet to be answered in a compelling way, though some evidence on both sides can be found. Other potential mechanisms exist, one of which we've already alluded to: the cumulative stress model, associated with the often-lengthy legal proceedings. We've made a previous case for the biological and psychological influences of chronic stress on pain (and will do so again below), and believe this is likely a strong explanatory mechanism for the association with the medicolegal process. Another is the constant questioning about their pain that occurs at every doctor, physical therapist, chiropractor, independent evaluator, and lawyer's visit (for both the defense and prosecution) that provides a 'wobbly' foundation on which healing can occur. It should also be noted that while litigation is most commonly initiated to seek compensation for lost income, the process itself can also be tremendously expensive, and once a case has been initiated, the system does not allow much space for recovery to occur lest the injured person risk losing the case and have to bear the full burden of the proceedings themselves. Whether you choose to consider this phenomenon 'intentional exaggeration' is no doubt a matter of personal opinions, though we would offer an alternative explanation: that the personal injury litigation system in many countries is based on outdated understandings of pain, injury, and suffering, and as a result the patients seeking justice find themselves forced to play by rules that do not reflect the reality or complexity of their situation.

Whether intentional or not, we will not argue against the presence of an association between medicolegal involvement and ratings of pain severity. The very invisible nature of most pain conditions means these cases often come down to expert opinion, the likeability of the plaintiff and the sympathy they have been able to generate in those making the judgement (i.e. judge or jury). What's more is that expert witnesses are bound by burdens of truth when in fact there remains few diagnostic options for many pain conditions by which to tip the scales of justice. It truly comes down to their own impressions, experiences, interpretations of the patient, interpretations of the available clinical notes from any number of healthcare providers (all of whom likely 'speak a different language'), the patient's history, including pre-existing health status, results on imaging tests, reports of crash parameters, perhaps even their relationship with the attorneys on both sides. From all of this, the expert is asked to opine as to whether it is more likely true than not the patient has the level of impairment and disability that they report. We encourage readers to reflect upon other potential mechanisms to explain the phenomena beyond assuming everyone will, in fact, get better with a pile of $100 bills.

Pre-trauma adversity

We've left this domain for last as it will likely include all of the prior ones in some form or another. To start this mechanistic conversation, we first posit the following: no trauma or pain occurs in a vacuum. That is, we all bring our own baggage, shaped by prior life experiences, current physical and emotional status, and the cacophony of experiences that occur immediately before and after a trauma. This is one reason why animal models are not easily translatable to humans – while we can induce stress and anxiety and any

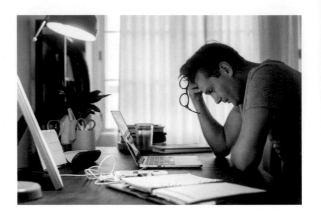

number of health conditions in mice, those mice do not go home after the trauma to pay their bills, prepare dinner, and care for their children or aging parents. They do not field phone calls from creditors, argue with their spouse about spending habits, or worry about that weird rash on their child's stomach. Where animal studies, with their tightly controlled methods, can provide considerable information on processes of disease, they cannot explain the messiness of what it means to be a human in a complex sociocultural environment. As has become abundantly clear to this point, we believe one strong mechanism of pain ratings is the cumulative physiological and psychological burden of chronic stress. Stress science is every bit as complex as that of the social determinants of health, so once again this is at best a cursory overview of decades of research.

Chronic stress has far-reaching effects: whether due to the physiological load of persistent HPA axis activity and the long-term effects of hypercortisolism, or the vagal connection between gut and brain, or the disturbed sleep, lethargy, fatigue, and general lack of recreational activity that occurs during times of high stress, to the atrophied dopaminergic, opioidergic, and serotonergic brain pathways that would otherwise help to stabilize mood in times of relative joy, there are any number of these or other pathways that may explain the physiological association between stress and pain following trauma. Emotional resilience is also limited during times of heightened or chronic stress, and optimism can be hard to come by. Perhaps not surprisingly, negative expectations of a positive outcome are a strong predictor of a poor recovery, possibly illuminating a link between chronic stress and recovery. Any clinician who considers every patient as simply a data point from population-based research is bound for a dissatisfying result, as every person is different regardless of how representative the sampling approach of that study may have been or the rigor of the randomization process. We suggest that it is that messiness and uniqueness of humans that may be an important explanation for the inability of traditional randomized clinical trials to find much in the way of significant impact of many pain-related interventions.

Additionally, we must address pre-trauma stressors. Work in our labs and many others around the world are exploring the potential impacts of early childhood adversity on adult health status and outcomes. Considerable research in both animals and humans has now accumulated providing compelling evidence that, despite the well-worn adage, time does not heal all wounds. Some very large-scale cohort studies, such as the Adverse Childhood Experiences (ACE) study run through a collaboration between the American health maintenance organization Kaiser Permanente and the U.S. Centers for Disease Control (CDC) have shown that cumulative experiences of trauma in childhood lead to greater likelihood and impact of chronic health conditions, including chronic pain, in adulthood (Felitti et al., 1998). It should likely come as no surprise that experiences of trauma in childhood influence one's reaction to trauma in adulthood, though potentially surprising is that this does not appear to be a solely psychological phenomenon. In fact, many have found that the experience of,

or exposure to, significant childhood trauma leads to observable *methylation* of key genetic markers that are also associated with resilience to health stressors later in life; a field of study that has become known as 'epigenetics'. In other words, childhood trauma, including witnessing OR experiencing sexual, physical, and/or emotional abuse, neglect, poverty, violence, crime, significant health threats, family disruption, or substance abuse, leads to observable changes in the genes of the child that appear to have lifelong effects on the physiological reactions to subsequent health or other threats. The going hypothesis is that these changes then lead one to be more vulnerable to experiences causing pain or disease throughout adulthood. In fact, a fairly compelling body of evidence suggests that these early traumas can occur while the child is still in the womb, where it is the stress experienced by the mother that affects the offspring. And even more interesting is that, being a genetic change, this influence of trauma on health can persist across generations, now termed *intergenerational trauma*.

Stop us if we've said this before, but humans are wonderfully 'messy' creatures.

These are just some of the phenomena that very likely have real impact on the number a patient will assign to their pain when you ask them to rate it between zero and ten, yet the mechanisms to explain each, and the knowledge of how to modify treatment as a result, is currently theoretical at best. The primary reason for us raising these issues is to ensure we do not forget about equality and fairness in management of a patient's unique experience with pain. We've just laid out considerable evidence to suggest that women, ethnocultural minorities, those of lower socioeconomic backgrounds or lower education, on average, will report greater pain severity than their more socially, educationally, and financially privileged counterparts. However, epidemiological and practice evidence also indicates that those less advantaged groups are also less likely to receive adequate pain management and to experience stigma from their healthcare providers. There is of course no easy solution to addressing inequality, be it in healthcare or otherwise, but we hope that by raising awareness, readers will be encouraged to spend a bit of time reflecting on their own biases and practices and recognize those times when their treatment decisions have been influenced more by personal than clinical factors.

Distinguishing features

The focus here is to identify those patients for whom a socioenvironmental driver is the *primary* driver, or at least a disproportionately strong driver, of their pain.

To start we can offer signs that would lead you *away* from identifying socioenvironmental influences as a primary driver. These can largely be found in the prior chapters of this book. For example, pain that is clearly and predictably linked to specific postures or movements would point you in a different direction. Consistent signs of allodynia or hyperalgesia, problems with things like two-point discrimination or laterality recognition, a clear history of a peripheral nerve lesion, ineffective conditioned pain modulation, or strong evidence of psychopathology would all logically point to other domains as *primary* drivers. Even then of course, it would be too reductionistic to suggest that social drivers are not also influencing pain ratings, but we need to put boundaries around this somehow.

The clear signs leading you towards this domain as a primary or strong driver will largely need to be disclosed by the patient themselves. These could include job dissatisfaction or workplace harassment, financial instability, experiences of interpersonal or intimate partner violence (either as an adult or during childhood), unsafe or non-permanent shelter, living in a disadvantaged or unsafe neighborhood, or those without an adaptive social support network. Other things are more obvious and should not be used to stereotype a patient, but rather identified in the interest of cultural safety and equality, including things like sex, gender orientation, ethnic background, education, and being involved in litigation. Again, we cannot stress this enough: none of these should be used by a clinician to judge the legitimacy of a patient's complaint. Rather, clinicians should consider what they know about the patient and how those things may lead to differences in patient-provider expectations, values, beliefs, or needs in terms of pain management and rehabilitation to build patient-centered and collaborative care plans.

Prognostic value

Much of this work is in its infancy but is rapidly evolving. Some readers will be aware of the concepts of blue flags (perceived work barriers) and black flags (actual work barriers) in predicting return to work (Shaw et al., 2009). The most evidentiary support for the usefulness of the blue and black flags in the musculoskeletal field can be found in low back pain. That is, a perception of job dissatisfaction, toxic interpersonal work relationships, or physical demands that are too far beyond the injured worker's capacity to perform, appear to be predictors of unsuccessful return to work. The Fear-Avoidance Beliefs Questionnaire (FABQ) has a subscale dedicated to work barriers, best conceptualized as 'blue flags', that has fair evidence to support its prognostic value in acute low back pain. Spousal responses to patient reports of pain have also been shown to predict poor recovery, most commonly measured using a tool called the Spousal Response Inventory (SRI, not to be confused with the *Satisfaction and Recovery Index*). Raichle and colleagues explored the ability of SRI scores to predict pain reports and behaviors in a sample of 94 people with chronic pain. They found that patient reports of

🔧	**Suggested evidence for triangulation: socioenvironmental domain**	

Test domains	Findings	Shift in likelihood
Screening tools	There are a number of such tools that exist, and providers are encouraged to at least search them out and review the items so that they are prepared to hear potential issues as they arise. These include the Injustice Experience Questionnaire (IEQ), the Gender Roles and Expectations of Pain scale (GREP), the Pain Catastrophizing Scale – significant other version (PCS-so, completed by the significant other *about* the patient), the Adverse Childhood Experiences questionnaire (ACE, should only be administered by those familiar with its use and interpretation), and the Spousal Response Inventory. Tools to measure concepts related to work satisfaction, decision-making power, and functional capacity needs are plentiful and can be found easily online.	++
Symptom behavior	The most likely sign here will be pain that appears to fluctuate in accordance with contextual factors. That could include pain that is worse when at home or in the presence of a spouse (in the case of partner violence), pain that worsens as the patient is preparing to return to work (in the case of workplace problems), or other patterns such as pain around bill payment or tax time, pain that worsens in the presence of lawyers or when in the presence of other healthcare providers with whom the patient has a poor relationship. None of these should be *assumed* to indicate intentional exaggeration, but all would warrant further exploration by a trained member of the circle of care.	+
Palpation	If the *primary* driver is due to adverse socioenvironmental influences, then there should arguably be no consistent palpatory findings. However, in the case that pain *is* being exaggerated or is being used as a defense mechanism to protect the patient from returning to an adverse environment, you may identify consistent areas of increased pain sensitivity. There have been a number of tests developed over the years that are intended to identify this type of biased pain reporting including some that involve repeated palpation or pressure algometry. Most of these are more commonly used by neuropsychiatrists in the medicolegal context, and most of which possess questionable measurement and discrimination properties.	Neutral
Quantitative sensory testing	As per palpation, many QST tests have at some point been explored for their value as 'objective' pain measures to assess the validity of a patient's pain complaint, though in our opinion, as of this writing, no such tools truly fit that definition. However, the field is moving rapidly and we would say that if a clinician were really looking for pain that does not fit any of the other domains in this framework and decided to apply several such tests, including pressure, current, thermal and vibratory detection thresholds, nociceptive flexion withdrawal reflex testing, tests of conditioned pain modulation, and perhaps other more emerging tests (e.g. pupil constriction response, electrodermal response), then it is possible a sign indicating a strong socioenvironmental driver would emerge from integrating the results of several of these tests that do not consistently support any other driver. That is, inconsistent results are the positive sign here. We urge caution in this interpretation though.	+
Sensorimotor testing	Possibly, when used in conjunction with the QST tests above for further triangulation, *inconsistencies* in things like two-point discrimination, laterality, joint position sense error, postural sway or others *may* indicate that the primary pain drivers are external to the person, though this is quite speculative.	+
Mechanical testing	Evidence for triangulation when identifying pain with a primary socioenvironmental driver could come from a *lack* of consistent or predictable mechanical patterns of pain reproduction. As such, the contributing evidence is the non-mechanical pattern.	+

—*continued*—

Test domains	Findings	Shift in likelihood
	Suggested evidence for triangulation: socioenvironmental domain *continued*	
Cognitions	If a *primary* socioenvironmental driver is referring to those influences external to the person, then signs of maladaptive beliefs or cognitions of the person would not be evidence of this domain. Of course, it is *very* likely that those with strong external pressures will probably also endorse maladaptive thoughts about their pain, and this is the value of the radar plot: it allows both cognitive and socioenvironmental drivers to be present in the same person.	Neutral
Emotions	Very similar to the cognitions commentary: while negative emotional or mood status is likely to accompany things like external stressors or job dissatisfaction, in the absence of those external influences, negative affect in isolation would not provide evidence of a socioenvironmental driver.	Neutral
Socioenvironmental	Clinicians should develop their skills around sensitive and respectful questioning to explore external socioenvironmental influences that may be leading to a patient rating their pain as more severe. This is clearly the most telling set of evidence to identify a primary driver in this domain.	+++
Pathology	If a clinician were to argue that the primary driver of a patient's pain experience is socioenvironmental, then observable pathology would not be evidence thereof. Rather, pain in the absence of pathology is a stronger piece of evidence, though would be highly non-specific as this could also be evidence of any domain other than nociceptive or neuropathic. So, the evidence here is a *lack* of obvious lesion or pathology.	+

either overly solicitous spousal responses (too much of the 'don't you try doing that, I'll do it instead' type responses) or overly punitive responses (too much of the 'stop being such a wimp and get on with it' type responses) were both predictive of pain severity (Raichle et al., 2011). However, as these are all reported by the patient, both results using the FABQ and SRI may be better considered cognitive (patient's perceptions) than actual socioenvironmental influences. It's a bit of a muddy area.

An interesting example of socioenvironmental influences on prognosis can be found in the work of Ulirsch and colleagues, who conducted a moderator analysis of their prior findings of a genetic vulnerability to persistent pain following road traffic collisions

(Ulirsch et al., 2014). In their first study they identified certain genes that, based on the set of alleles (certain amino acid pairings) present, could classify people into 'high pain vulnerable' or 'low pain vulnerable' genotypes. That was interesting enough on its own, but as a follow-up they asked the question of whether genotype interacts with social context to either increase or decrease risk, especially in those who are genetically vulnerable. They found that zip code, as a proxy for socioeconomic status (SES), interacted with genotype in such a way that the magnitude of risk associated with the 'high pain vulnerable' genotype was influenced by SES; those who were genetically vulnerable but from a higher SES were more protected against persistent pain than were those who were both genetically vulnerable *and* lived in an area with lower SES. This is an example of what is referred to as a 'gene x environment' interaction and is an important reminder that risk and prognosis is never simple, but is a complex interplay of personal and contextual factors in every person.

In 2013, we conducted a systematic review and meta-analysis of prognostic factors following acute whiplash, and found that lower education appeared to have some prognostic value, though the state of the evidence was not good enough (and arguably still is not) to tell us whether lower education *causes* poor recovery, or as we've described above, is operating as a proxy for some other confounding variable such as health literacy, cognitive resilience, alternative opportunities for employment, and access to care. In a subsequent study we have also found that those participants who describe more life stressors (not related to the trauma) either recently or in early life also had more complex clinical presentations and were less likely to report full recovery six months later. Again, we cannot opine with confidence on the causal nature of these findings, including which is the chicken and which is the egg, and whether intervening in any way would reduce the likelihood of chronic pain. However, we can say with confidence that, on average, those people who have lived under a greater burden of life stress, be it due to SES, education, housing, interpersonal trauma, or ethnic, religious, or sex/gender-based marginalization, are more likely than their otherwise privileged counterparts to experience persistent pain.

Intervention strategies

Intervention strategies here will be as varied and potentially ambiguous as the nature of the socioenvironmental factors themselves. What would be an intervention strategy for lower educational background or lower socioeconomic status? Send patients back to school? Cut them a check? Unreasonable would

be an understatement here. Instead, our position on all of these socioenvironmental factors based on the current state of knowledge in the field, is that all should be considered and explored as appropriate with patients, and providers should be willing to *adapt their other intervention strategies accordingly.* Does the patient understand your educational intervention? Can they afford the resources (medications, gym equipment, adaptive housing) that you've recommended? Are your treatment recommendations relevant to them in terms of gender, age, religious, or ethnocultural background? For those who have been the victims of interpersonal violence, is it reasonable or appropriate for you to think you can touch them to provide a manual treatment? If they are the victims of workplace harassment, how might that affect their motivation to adhere to your return-to-work-focused treatment plan? Clinicians are strongly encouraged to explore these influences on a patient's pain experience to the extent that it is reasonable and appropriate to do so, and to develop their skills in listening for subtle cues in a patient's story or watching for them during an intervention session, and to be prepared to act on them when they arise. It reminds us of the words of Sir Winston Churchill:

Courage is what it takes to stand up and speak; courage is also what it takes to sit down and listen.

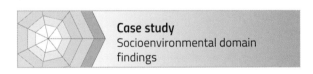

Case study
Socioenvironmental domain findings

Returning to our case of Sean, we are primarily interested in those 'other' external or contextual factors, such as financial, job, or interpersonal stress, housing and community, culture and religion, isolation, past experiences, family, medical, and medicolegal influences on a person's pain experience (either the experience of the pain, or the expression of the pain – the distinction does not currently matter). Through appropriate and sensitive questioning, Sean describes himself as a dedicated father to his two children, stating that he himself had a rough childhood and that he vowed 'not to be like my father'. He is now in a stable relationship with a common-law partner, living in a comfortable and safe neighborhood, and mostly enjoys his job despite the high stakes involved. As the executive assistant, he actually has considerable control over his boss's (and therefore his own) schedule, which allows him to enjoy greater flexibility than most in his company. He describes his relationship with his doctor as very good, and so far, feels that his insurance company has been more supportive than punitive. He describes many of the same stresses as most middle-class families in your region, but thanks to some wise investing and his partner's income he is not yet concerned about a temporary loss of his own income, though would become more concerned if the recovery drags on. So far, his boss has been supportive

of some time off work, and his company health benefits are good enough to cover at least most of his current course of therapy.

While there are some minor potential issues in Sean's story, including his allusion to a difficult childhood, there are no significant pieces of evidence here that would lead us to triangulate a strong socioenvironmental driver of Sean's pain experience. This may well change with time however, especially if the recovery does not go smoothly (a high possibility given his initial presentation). So, we should be sure to check back with him about any mounting external stressors over time. For now, we'll leave the relative contribution from this domain fairly low. (Fig. 12.1)

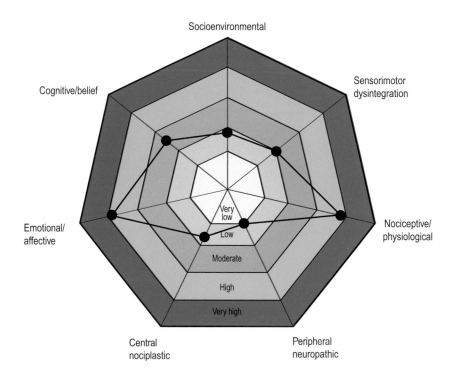

Figure 12.1
Sean's radar plot continues to take shape. Based on the socioenvironmental domain findings, this driver has been kept at 'low' probability.

References

Ahn, H., Weaver, M., Lyon, D. E., et al., 2017. Differences in clinical pain and experimental pain sensitivity between Asian Americans and whites with knee osteoarthritis. *The Clinical Journal of Pain* 33 (2):174–80.

Felitti, V. J., Anda, R. F., Nordenberg, D., et al., 1998. Relationship of childhood abuse and household dysfunction to many of the leading causes of death in adults. The Adverse Childhood Experiences (ACE) Study. *American Journal of Preventive Medicine* 14 (4):245–58.

Ferrari, R., Kwan, O., Russell, A. S., et al., 1999. The best approach to the problem of whiplash? One ticket to Lithuania, please. *Clinical and Experimental Rheumatology* 17 (3):321–6.

Fuentes, M., Hart-Johnson, T., Green, C. R., 2007. The association among neighborhood socioeconomic status, race and chronic pain in black and white older adults. *Journal of the National Medical Association* 99 (10): 1160–9.

Hadler, N. M., 1996. If you have to prove you are ill, you can't get well. The object lesson of fibromyalgia. *Spine* 21 (20):2397–400.

Raichle, K. A., Romano, J. M., Jensen, M. P., 2011. Partner responses to patient pain and well behaviors and their relationship to patient pain behavior, functioning, and depression. *Pain* 152 (1): 82–8.

Shaw, W. S., van der Windt, D. A., Main, C. J., et al., 2009. Early patient screening and intervention to address individual-level occupational factors ('blue flags') in back disability. *Journal of Occupational Rehabilitation* 19 (1):64–80.

Spearing, N. M., Connelly, L. B., 2011. Whiplash and the compensation hypothesis. *Spine* 36 (25 Suppl):S303-8.

Spearing, N. M., Connelly, L. B., Gargett, S., et al., 2012a. Does injury compensation lead to worse health after whiplash? A systematic review. *Pain* 153 (6):1274–82.

Spearing, N. M., Gyrd-Hansen, D., Pobereskin, L. H., et al., 2012b. Are people who claim compensation 'cured by a verdict'? A longitudinal study of health outcomes after whiplash. *Journal of Law and Medicine* 20 (1):82–92.

Ulirsch, J. C., Weaver, M. A., Bortsov, A. V., et al., 2014. No man is an island: living in a disadvantaged neighborhood influences chronic pain development after motor vehicle collision. *Pain* 155 (10):2116–23.

13

The Sensorimotor Dysintegration Domain

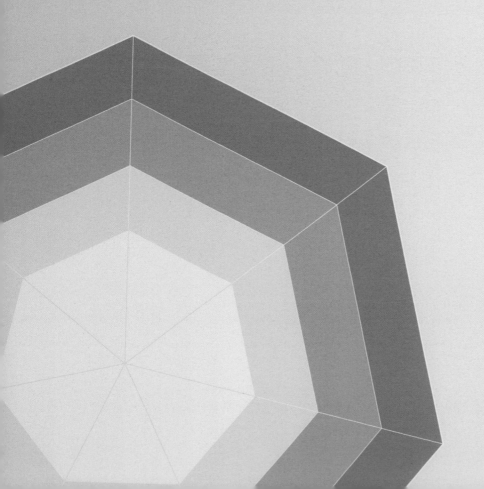

Proposed mechanisms

Integrating and processing information from multiple external and internal sources to form perception about the world around us, and our perceived and actual status within it, is a key function of the brain. This ability forms one half of an active feedback loop allowing humans and other life to accomplish pretty impressive tasks, like quickly locating environmental cues and threats, remaining engaged in a conversation with a friend in a noisy environment, navigating a room in the dark without bumping into things, or maintaining an upright posture without falling over. Taking the latter as an example, the ability for humans to stand upright is nothing short of a miraculous integration of moment-to-moment processing and comparison of information coming from diverse sources such as the touch- (pressure) sensitive afferents on the soles of our feet, through the tension sensors in our lower extremity and trunk muscles, the pattern of light and lines hitting the rods and cones on the backs of our eyeballs, to the subtle bending of almost imperceptibly small hairs bathed in a fluidic environment of the semicircular canals located within our inner ears (Fig. 13.1). Even the subtlest of changes to any one of these can result in an immediate action of magnitude and purpose that is capable of maintaining bipedal upright posture without falling over.

Integration and interpretation of diverse information is arguably one of the most important functions of the brain, which is constantly sampling from countless sensors in our body to maintain a state of relative 'normal'. Blood pressure, heart rate, glucose levels, body temperature, muscle tone, and nervous system sensitivity are just some examples of the

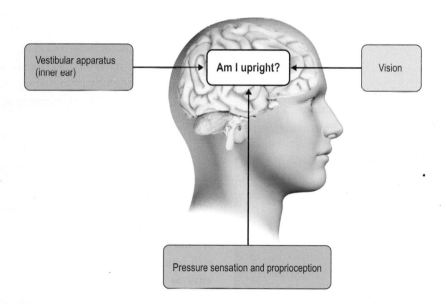

Figure 13.1

Simple schematic of an example of sensorimotor integration. The brain receives information from multiple sources, including the eyes (Is the horizon horizontal? Are the corners of the walls vertical?), the vestibular apparatus in the inner ear (sort of like the accelerometer and gyroscope in your smartphone), and input from various skin and musculoskeletal afferents, including the skin on the bottom of your feet (Is the sensation of pressure changing location?) and the tension sensors in your muscles and tendons. These are all integrated on a time scale of milliseconds to help the brain answer the question 'Am I upright?' If the answer is clearly 'yes', no change in action is required. If the answer is clearly 'no' then motor nerves are activated to regain balance. If the answer is 'not sure' or 'conflicting information', the system may not be sure what to do, resulting in sense of vertigo or nausea. The latter would be an example of sensorimotor dysintegration.

numerous physiological processes that must remain within fairly narrow limits for humans and animals to function and survive. This process of maintaining some state of 'normality', commonly referred to as *homeostasis*, is critical for survival, and deviation from it is often the first warning sign that something might be amiss. A foreign invader will likely lead to elevated white blood cells; elevated or lowered body temperature may indicate an environmental threat to be addressed; or a sudden burst of activity from high-threshold nociceptive afferents may indicate actual or potential tissue damage is occurring. The brain needs to be able to rapidly (within milliseconds) receive, integrate, interpret, and if needed, act upon such information to ensure your survival and ongoing function. But what if the information coming into the brain paints an incomplete, or even contradictory, picture? What does the brain do – or not do – then?

The *sensorimotor dysintegration* domain is characterized by a pain experience that is driven by this type of discord in information arriving from various body sensors. Consider for example, a situation in which the information arriving from your optic sensors (your eyes) is sending a message that your head is perfectly positioned between your shoulders and is plumb (upright) compared to the cues in your environment (such as the horizon or corners of intersecting walls). Yet, the information arriving from the muscle spindles and Golgi tendon organs (GTOs) that are in rich abundance in your neck muscles are sending a message that the right middle scalenus muscle is slightly stretched (more tension) while the left is slightly relaxed (less tension) indicating your head is in fact slightly side-flexed to the left relative to your thorax (Fig. 13.2). As far as we can tell, and to no doubt oversimplify a tremendously complex set of events, the brain does not like this type of conflict. At the risk of anthropomorphizing (and being admittedly dualistic), the brain, meant to be the constant foreman of your body status, is now unable to determine whether

your head is upright or slightly tilted. As a result, it has lost its comfort in detecting threat and may choose to err on the side of caution, raising alarms of actual or potential tissue damage.

The prefix 'dys' comes from the Greek meaning 'wrong' or 'abnormal'. This is different from 'dis' (as in disintegration) meaning 'apart', 'away' or 'undo'. So, in this context, *dysintegration* refers to a lack of coherence or integration.

It has been hypothesized that this type of dysintegration could be a primary driver for several chronic pain conditions such as phantom limb pain, complex regional pain syndrome, chronic whiplash associated disorders, post-concussion syndrome, or central post-stroke pain. The theory, admittedly somewhat difficult to test, goes something like this: the brain is constantly sampling from the billions of sensors in your body in the interest of maintaining homeostasis of the whole organism. Part of that will be periodic 'scanning' of the boundaries of your body in space. That is, as the theory goes, your brain knows where your body ends (part of interoception) and your 'outside' (environment) begins. It does this by frequently sampling from the end organs (Pacinian corpuscles, Ruffini endings, Meissner's corpuscles, free nerve endings, and others) embedded within your skin, muscles, and tendons, and comparing that against a lifetime of archived information that has provided a pretty clear *somatotopic representation* of your body 'schema', or 'corporeal representation' (Berlucchi & Aglioti, 2010). As Berlucchi and Aglioti reviewed, these concepts are not universally embraced in the scientific or medical communities, though few concepts are. However, it would explain why, after years (decades) of 'all clear out here on the periphery!' messages being returned when the brain sends out a call for a status update, that when presented with

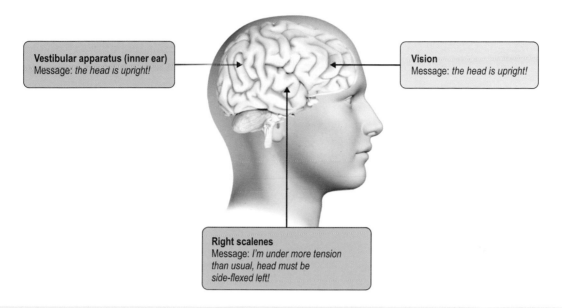

Vestibular apparatus (inner ear)
Message: *the head is upright!*

Vision
Message: *the head is upright!*

Right scalenes
Message: *I'm under more tension than usual, head must be side-flexed left!*

Figure 13.2
A simple diagrammatic representation of sensorimotor dysintegration in neck pain. Here, the vestibular apparatus and eyes are both providing information to the brain indicating that the head is perfectly upright. Conversely, perhaps as a result of trauma, the muscular tension sensors (muscle spindles, Golgi tendon organs) in the right anterior, middle, and posterior scalenes are indicating that muscle is under more tension than normal, suggesting that the head may in fact be side-flexed to the left. Under this theory, the discordant information from different sources leads to experiences that may be interpreted as pain (or nausea, dizziness, increased protective spasm or 'guarding', etc.).

a sudden 'dead phone line', the result is an alarm of potential trauma and danger. Of course, even without peripheral input, that 'body schema' map still knows where the limb is *supposed* to be, and therefore the resulting unpleasant sensory and emotional experience is felt *as though* it is arising from the limb that, in the case of phantom limb pain, is no longer even there.

Now it would be a mighty problematic rehabilitation journey for a patient suffering from phantom head or neck pain, however, there is evidence accumulating to suggest that some people with chronic regional or widespread pain conditions may also show signs consistent with these other 'central sensorimotor dysintegration' drivers. For example, a relatively simple, but impactful, study by pain researcher Lorimer Moseley led to some rather interesting and potentially important results (Moseley, 2008). Dr. Moseley presented six participants with chronic low back pain a line drawing of the outline of a body, but with the lower back part missing. They were asked to complete the missing part of the drawing by adding in lines to indicate how they perceived their back (how it feels, rather than how it looks). They were also asked to indicate on the same drawing the boundaries of their pain by drawing a rough circle around it. Finally, the participants were requested to lie on their stomachs to undergo a test called 'two-point discrimination' at the approximate level of each vertebral segment of the lumbar spine. The two-point discrimination (2PD) test requires participants to indicate whether they perceive the two points of a set of calipers as two distinct points, or as just one point. The smaller the number the better, in that it means better tactile acuity, and 2PD itself has been recently endorsed as a means to tap into cortical reorganization of the body schema. Figure 13.3 shows the somewhat unanticipated results of this very interesting study. First, it became obvious from the drawings that the people in this study, each of which

had a complex history of chronic low back pain, also perceived the boundaries of their lower backs in a very distorted and inaccurate way, suggesting that their body schemas of the painful area were also distorted. This was corroborated by the 2PD findings in those same areas, suggesting that some component of their pain experience may be related to, or perhaps sustained by, discordant information arriving at the cortex and an inability of the brain to therefore get a handle on the true state of the tissues 'out there' on the periphery.

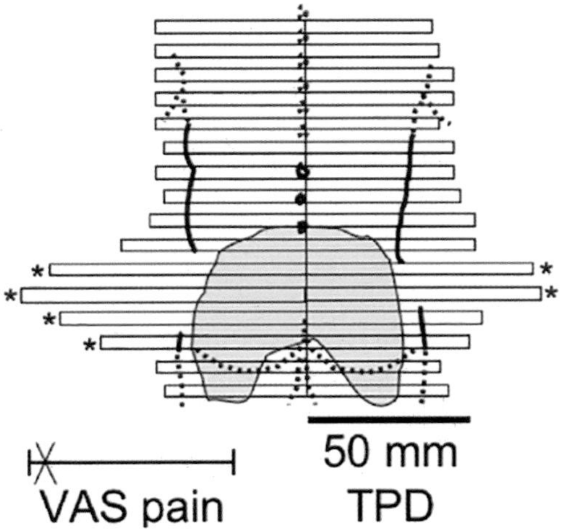

Similar phenomena can be seen in other body regions and through different modalities. Going back to our upright posture example earlier, Field and colleagues conducted a study exploring postural sway (the movement of the body's center of mass measured using a force platform during normal and balance-challenged standing) in people with *traumatic* and those with *non-traumatic* neck pain (Field et al., 2008). While both neck pain groups were more unsteady than people without neck pain, those with traumatic neck pain swayed a lot more than those with non-traumatic neck pain. They hypothesized that this may be due to damage to tissues in the neck that provide proprioceptive (relative tension/relaxation/compression) information to the brain to maintain upright posture, resulting in discordant information arriving at the brain. Focusing on a different mode of assessment, de Vries and colleagues systematically searched and synthesized the available evidence on *joint position sense error* (JPSE) in people with and without neck pain (de Vries et al., 2015). JPSE refers to the ability of a person to return their body part to a starting (usually neutral) position when their visual information is blocked (eyes closed or blindfolded). It is generally accepted that, at least when referring to head and neck movement and assuming the patient is seated, that realignment to a 'neutral' position is a result of visual input, the inner ear vestibular

Figure 13.3
Two-point discrimination (TPD) threshold, normal distribution of pain, and body image. TPD was assessed bilaterally at 16 levels, shown here superimposed over line drawings of the sense of physical self, or body image, of one patient with chronic back pain. Dotted lines formed the template given to patient. Solid lines are those added by the patient. Shaded area shows distribution of pain marked on a body chart by the patient prior to other assessments. Horizontal bars show the TPD threshold at each of 16 levels taken bilaterally. Asterisk denotes different to the mean TPD for that patient by more than three standard deviations. Note missing outlines of the back in the zone of this patient's usual pain. (With permission from Prof. G. Lorimer Moseley. Adapted from Moseley, 2008.)

apparatus and the proprioceptive information (spindles and GTOs) from the soft tissues. Take vision away and all the person is left with is what their vestibular apparatus and cervical proprioceptors are telling them. If one of those is damaged/injured/dysfunctional, identification of neutral (or any other position) is bound to be inaccurate. This is largely what de Vries found, and similar to postural sway, the effect was stronger in people with traumatic neck pain than those with non-traumatic (idiopathic) neck pain.

There are several other such examples that can be found in the field of chronic pain. Much of it has also been corroborated by fMRI evidence, showing that in people with different types of chronic pain, the somatotopic representation of the painful area on the cerebral cortex has been shifted, blurred, expanded, shrunk, or otherwise changed (see for example Hotz-Boendermaker et al., 2016; Flor, 2002; Apkarian et al., 2011). For our purposes, the domain of *sensorimotor dysintegration* can be taken to refer to any process involving the central nervous system's ability (or inability) to process, synthesize, and compare numerous sources of information *except* actual or potential tissue damage. The latter is reserved for the central nociplastic domain that has been covered on a different point, while sensorimotor will be reserved for touch, visual, proprioceptive, vestibular, and any other non-noxious sensory input that, when in disagreement with one another, can (we propose) function to drive or sustain a pain experience.

Distinguishing features

There are several possible clues that astute clinicians may pick up during a patient interaction that could raise the index of suspicion of a primary sensorimotor driver of pain. Given the evidence just described, the history or mechanism underlying their current complaint (e.g. trauma) could be a great first clue, but never in isolation, and not always occurring. Others

may include descriptions of the injured body part that do not appear to be consistent with reality, such as an insistence that the injured part is swollen, hot, or red, when the clinician can clearly see that none of those appears true. Reports from the patient of more frequently bumping into things when walking, tripping over even small bumps, or dropping things more than usual could all indicate that the patient is having difficulty integrating the boundaries of their body in relation to their environment, though more sinister causes of ataxia should also be explored here. Problems when reading that have emerged since the injury (most relevant to head/neck trauma) or reports of now being highly sensitive to light, noise, odor or temperature may indicate sensory processing problems. Unsteadiness when standing, feelings of dizziness (which again could be the result of any number of mechanisms so should be explored further), or difficulty performing even simple exercises correctly may indicate sensorimotor coordination deficits. Clinical tests may also be of value here, though none in isolation is likely sensitive enough to declare a sensorimotor dysintegration problem with high levels of confidence. Two-point discrimination (Fig. 13.4), laterality recognition (the ability to quickly scan a photograph of a living body and accurately determine whether the photo is showing a right or left hand, foot, neck, or back; Fig. 13.5), and joint position sense error (Fig. 13.6) may all have some value for tapping this domain. Triangulating findings will be key here, as many of these are at best coarse (low resolution) indicators of sensorimotor problems and are generally more sensitive than they are specific, but when several different ones point in the same direction, this strengthens confidence in a primary sensorimotor dysintegration driver.

Prognostic Value

According to the available scientific evidence, prognostic utility of any sensorimotor dysintegration test

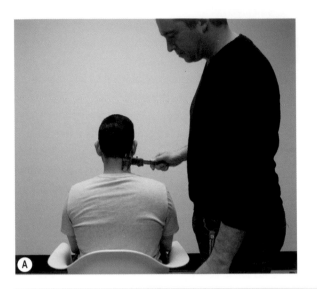

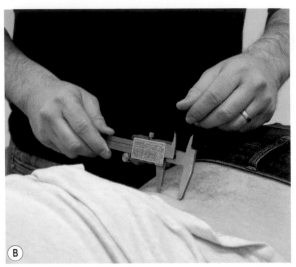

Figure 13.4
Examples of two-point discrimination (2PD) testing at the neck (**A**) and low back (**B**). In the most common protocol, simple calipers can be used that are touched to the skin just enough to cause an indent. The calipers are started at 0mm, and the patient is asked to indicate whether they perceive one point or two. The distance between the calipers is increased by 5mm and touched to the skin again. This continues until the patient perceives two points. Then the calipers are expanded an additional 2–3 cm, and the same process is conducted in reverse (decreasing distance between the calipers by 5mm each time). This ramp up/ramp down protocol can be repeated two or three times if precision is needed. Validity in the result is supported when the two-point threshold is within 5mm in both the ramp up and ramp down directions. A positive test would be a very different (e.g. >1 cm) 2PD threshold either between sides at the same level, or between the affected level and ones above and below it.

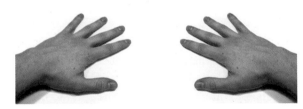

Figure 13.5
In a laterality judgement task, patients are shown pictures of the affected body part (e.g. hand, foot, shoulder, knee) and asked to make a judgement about whether they are looking at a right or left hand as quickly as possible. People with sensorimotor dysintegration problems are likely to make more errors when shown the affected side, or take longer making the decision.

in predicting the persistence or severity of chronic pain is largely unknown. Theoretically speaking, it does makes sense that, when identified even in the acute stage of an injury, those with greater signs of sensorimotor integration problems are less likely to recover quickly. However, this has largely been absent from musculoskeletal prognostic research to date. Wang and colleagues found that, of people undergoing lower limb nerve decompression for diabetic peripheral neuropathy, worse two-point discrimination before surgery was retained in their prediction models for worse pain relief after surgery (Wang et al., 2018). In a small study, Harvie and colleagues found that two-point discrimination

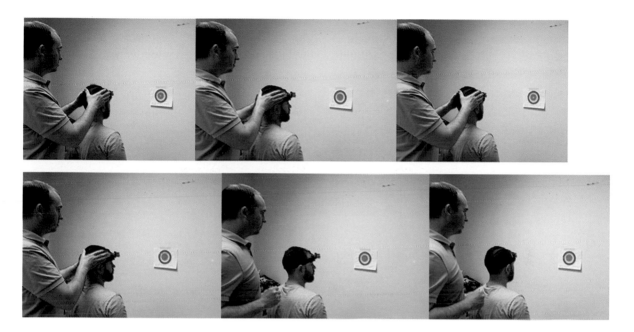

Figure 13.6
A sample test for joint position sense error (JPSE) of the neck. A target is placed on the wall 90 cm in front of the patient. The patient, wearing a head-mounted laser, is guided in feeling where the center position is on the target, then assisted as they rotate about 30 degrees and then back to center. On the second trial the clinician again guides the patient as they rotate 30 degrees, then removes the assistance and with eyes closed, the patient is asked to find the center point again. When a calibrated target is used (such as the one available for free at http://skillworks.biz/news/5995264), the amount of error (in degrees) can be easily recorded. More error = greater likelihood of a sensorimotor dysintegration problem.

measured at the neck in people with traumatic and non-traumatic neck pain was associated with higher pain intensity, but the prognostic value was not explored (Harvie et al., 2018). There are other limited examples of associations between sensorimotor dysintegration indicators and pain intensity (see for example the 2008 Moseley study in the proposed mechanisms section), but this is clearly an area ripe for further research.

Intervention strategies

Given the variety in sensorimotor tests available, intervention options can be quite varied. Much of it remains in the theoretical domain as there are very few clinical trials to lean on. However, in following the APT framework, this represents fertile ground for creativity for intervention options based on the specifics of your assessment findings. Increased (abnormal) joint position sense error may lead you towards interventions in which patients try to trace lines or shapes on a wall with a laser beam on their heads or perhaps novel uses of virtual reality technologies could be of help here. Two-point discrimination may improve following manual interventions focused on neural dynamics ('nerve flossing') in the upper limb in people with carpal tunnel syndrome (Wolny et al., 2016) or with electrotherapeutic (e.g. TENS) treatment. Other approaches to improving tactile acuity and two-point discrimination have been investigated to varying effectiveness, including drawing of letters on the lower back and providing feedback on the accuracy of patient guesses of what letter was drawn (Gutknecht et al., 2015), or wearing pads with small embedded vibratory motors over the skin and training patients to discriminate between the location and magnitude of the vibration (Stronks et al., 2017).

	Suggested evidence for triangulation: sensorimotor domain	
Test domains	**Findings**	**Shift in likelihood**
Screening tools	Self-report screening tools are rare here, though at least two exist. The first, called the Fremantle Back Awareness Questionnaire (FreBAQ; Wand et al., 2014) is intended for use in low back pain. The initial development study did show that patients with chronic LBP performed worse (median score of 11 vs. 0 for controls). An off-shoot of that has been created for the knee called the Fremantle Knee Awareness Questionnaire, available in Japanese only (FreKAQ-J; Nishigami et al., 2017). Known groups (discriminative) validity for the knee questionnaire has yet to be established. However, drawing on Moseley's work, one reasonable approach would be to provide patients with an incomplete line drawing of a body, where the painful region is missing, and ask them to complete the drawing as they perceive that region. This may provide clues, and strengthens our earlier arguments in favor of including some kind of body diagram as a 'go to' tool.	+ (low back pain only)
Symptom behavior	It will be difficult to identify any consistent symptom behaviors, including time of day, association with easing/aggravating activities, quality, or clearly delineated pain locations/boundaries. With the possible exception of pain that increases while reading, driving, in bright light, or when walking through the perfume section of a department store for example, the presence of *consistent* mechanical symptom behaviors would reduce the confidence in sensorimotor dysintegration.	Neutral to slight +
Palpation	Pain with a primary sensorimotor dysintegration driver is unlikely to be associated with palpation of known anatomical structures. It could be argued that the presence of trigger points (taut bands that refer pain when compressed and 'snap' when strummed under the fingers) may be associated with sensorimotor dysintegration inasmuch as increased muscle tone or peripheral motor facilitation may be a side effect of the brain's inability to accurately sample the tissues, but this would be so non-specific as to provide largely neutral evidence for this domain.	Neutral
Quantitative sensory testing	Pain-related QST measures, such as pressure pain or cold pain detection thresholds, should remain in the nociceptive, peripheral neuropathic, and central nociplastic domains. However, it is possible that non-pain related measures, such as current or vibration perception thresholds may be present in those with a primary sensorimotor dysintegration problem. Equally of course, those may also indicate small or large fiber neuropathy, so the value of any QST in identifying this domain as a primary driver is limited.	+

Suggested evidence for triangulation: sensorimotor domain *continued*

Test domains	Findings	Shift in likelihood
Sensorimotor testing	By definition, these are the clinical tests most likely to identify pain with a primary sensorimotor dysintegration driver. Work completed to date suggests that none of these *in isolation* is a definitive indicator of this driver, but three or more all suggesting a similar mechanism raises suspicion considerably. These include two-point discrimination (accuracy and acuity in identifying two contact points over one), laterality recognition (ability to quickly and accurately determine the laterality of the body part being viewed), joint position sense error (ability to nominate a neutral or starting position of a joint or joint complex), postural sway (the magnitude and behavior of the center of mass during standing usually done on a force platform and with increasing balance challenges), graphesthesia (ability to perceive and identify the shapes, such as letters, being traced on the injured body part when visual input is unavailable), smooth pursuit neck torsion test (ability to follow a finger with the eyes when the head is turned to the left or right (only relevant to neck pain)), or motor control tests (ability to 'correctly' perform movements or exercises of varying complexity when performed with the injured body part (see Luomajoki et al., 2008 for examples)). Ehrenbrust-off and colleagues conducted a recent systematic review that highlighted the relatively early stage of development of many such tests with focus on low back pain (Ehrenbrusthoff et al., 2018). Those conducted on other parts of the body (e.g. neck, limbs) generally show some value but considerable measurement error. As such, triangulation across tests is critical for identifying this driver.	+++
Mechanical testing	A clear mechanical pattern of symptoms would be evidence against a strong sensorimotor dysintegration driver, though clinicians should be cautious in their interpretation of mechanical or movement-based tests where tissue proprioceptors or, in the case of the neck, vestibular apparatus may be implicated, as movement of those regions may well result in increased pain. However, and this is critical, the presence of a pattern of pain provocation that is in keeping with known biomechanical (arthrokinetic or kinematic) principles would be evidence *against* sensorimotor dysintegration as the primary driver.	+ (when negative)
Cognitions	Not associated with this domain.	Neutral
Emotions	Not associated with this domain.	Neutral
Socioenviron-mental	Not associated with this domain.	Neutral
Pathology	The existence of clear musculoskeletal lesions on diagnostic testing that are obviously associated with the presentation of pain would be evidence against the sensorimotor dysintegration domain. However, if a diagnostician were able to conduct intraneural conduction integrity tests in, say, a type Ia or type II (muscle spindle) afferent, they may see impaired conduction. This would be highly unlikely to yield useable results with current diagnostic technologies.	Neutral

Motor control training has a long history in rehabilitation and has largely demonstrated some value in the lower back and neck, though the effect sizes of most interventions tend to be small (Saragiotto et al., 2016). Mirror box therapy, motor imagery, and laterality recognition training have been tested in people with phantom limb pain (Reinersmann et al., 2010) or complex regional pain syndrome (Moseley, 2004) and have shown some value in managing pain and improving the sensorimotor integration deficits. Patients who have difficulty identifying the boundaries of their bodies in space may benefit from manual contact therapies, though the mechanisms are unlikely to be biomechanical, but rather neurophysiological as the skin is rich with touch sensitive afferents. Drawing attention to those body parts may help address what has in the past been referred to as a quasi 'semi-neglect' of the painful body region in some people.

When using manual therapies for reasons of sensorimotor re-integration rather than biomechanical joint motion restoration, movement specificity (e.g. applying force to a specific joint in a specific direction) is a less important consideration than is the use of large contact surfaces and usually lighter pressures.

In almost all cases, any single intervention alone is unlikely to be of value, and when successful, the effects may be more relevant for the specific modality being trained than things like pain or function overall. However, pain with a primary sensorimotor dysintegration domain as the driver does tend to lend itself to somewhat imaginative interventions, and we anticipate further work in this domain to be rapidly forthcoming.

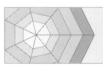

Case study
Sensorimotor dysintegration
domain findings

We return to our case of Sean one last time, to explore the possibility that other sensorimotor integration problems could be contributing to his experience of pain, headache, or other symptoms. From the initial interview we've already learned that he is describing troubles with eye fatigue and attending to different parts of his visual field. Whether these could be signs of a mild brain injury (e.g. concussion) or possibly a vestibulo-ocular integration or cervico-ocular proprioception problem is currently unknown and may be areas for further exploration. There are many directions we could take here to explore function of the cranial nerves, vestibular apparatus (semicircular canals), and cervical or whole-body proprioception/awareness. For the purposes of our case, we'll have Sean perform a few additional targeted tests.

The first is joint position sense error, where a head-mounted laser beam and wall-mounted target are used to determine how well Sean is able to nominate a neutral head/neck position with his eyes closed after we passively move his neck away from neutral (but within his painful limitations). We'll also conduct some two-point discrimination testing, and some ocular convergence/divergence testing. Finally, we'll have Sean stand in a tandem-standing (toe-to-heel) stance with his eyes open and eyes closed and observe how well he's able to maintain his upright posture when visual input is removed in this small base-of-support position. While 'normal' performance on most of these tests is not clear, a combination of poor performance across tests would be evidence for us to triangulate the relative contributions of sensorimotor dysintegration on his pain experience.

Despite the reports of eye fatigue and concentration, the in-clinic testing is largely normal for Sean. He is able to nominate a neutral cervical position fairly reliably with <5 degrees of error, there is no clear difference in two-point discrimination across cervical levels or sides, and eye tracking including convergence/divergence are within normal limits. On describing these results, Sean does state that even prior to the injury he had started to notice increased eye strain and some difficulties seeing clearly at a distance, and you suggest it may be

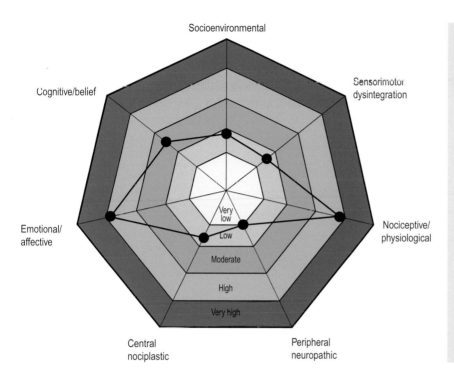

Figure 13.7
Sean's completed radar plot. The sensorimotor domain driver has been moved down slightly further in the 'low' probability range, and we can now clearly see that initial interventions should target the nociceptive/physiological and emotional drivers of Sean's pain experience.

time to visit an optometrist. For our purposes, there does not appear to be a strong sensorimotor component to Sean's pain experience.

After considering all domains then, Figure 13.7 shows Sean's final radar plot.

Summary

Here we can see that a tool like the radar plot, with a few well-informed questions and some rich clinical investigations can, in a fairly short period of time, identify the most appropriate *initial* targets for intervention in even a complex post-trauma case. Keep in mind however that as some of the initial primary drivers start to resolve (or persist), the relative contributions of others may increase, so periodic re-evaluation is highly recommended. By having this robust assessment procedure as a baseline, it should make future evaluations more targeted, efficient, and informative.

References

Apkarian, A. V., Hashmi, J. A., Baliki, M. N., 2011. Pain and the brain: specificity and plasticity of the brain in clinical chronic pain. *Pain* 152 (3 Suppl):S49–64.

Berlucchi, G., Aglioti, S. M., 2010. The body in the brain revisited. *Experimental Brain Research* 200 (1):25 35.

de Vries, J., Ischebeck, B. K., Voogt, L. P., et al., 2015. Joint position sense error in people with neck pain: A systematic review. *Manual Therapy* 20 (6):736–44.

Ehrenbrusthoff, K., Ryan, C. G., Grüneberg, C., et al., 2018. A systematic review and meta-analysis of the reliability and validity of sensorimotor measurement instruments in people with chronic low back pain. *Musculoskeletal Science and Practice* 35:73–83.

Field, S., Treleaven, J., Jull, G., 2008. Standing balance: a comparison between idiopathic and whiplash-induced neck pain. *Manual Therapy* 13 (3):183–91.

Flor, H., 2002. The modification of cortical reorganization and chronic pain by sensory feedback. *Applied Psychophysiology and Biofeedback* 27 (3):215–27.

Gutknecht, M., Mannig, A., Waldvogel, A., et al., 2015. The effect of motor control and tactile acuity training on patients with non-specific low back pain and movement control impairment. *Journal of Bodywork and Movement Therapies* 19 (4):722–31.

Harvie, D. S., Edmond-Hank, G., Smith, A. D., 2018. Tactile acuity is reduced in people with chronic neck pain. *Musculoskeletal Science and Practice* 33:61–6.

Hotz-Boendermaker, S., Marcar, V. L., Meier, M. L., et al., 2016. Reorganization in secondary somatosensory cortex in chronic low back pain patients. *Spine* 41 (11):E667–E673.

Luomajoki, H., Kool, J., de Bruin, E. D., et al., 2008. Movement control tests of the low back; evaluation of the difference between patients with low back pain and healthy controls. *BMC Musculoskeletal Disorders* 9 (1):170.

Moseley, G. L., 2004. Graded motor imagery is effective for long-standing complex regional pain syndrome: a randomised controlled trial. *Pain* 108 (1–2):192–8.

Moseley, G. L., 2008. I can't find it! Distorted body image and tactile dysfunction in patients with chronic back pain. *Pain* 140 (1):239–43.

Nishigami, T., Mibu, A., Tanaka, K., et al., 2017. Development and psychometric properties of knee-specific body-perception questionnaire in people with knee osteoarthritis: The Fremantle Knee Awareness Questionnaire. *PloS One* 12 (6):e0179225.

Reinersmann, A., Haarmeyer, G. S., Blankenburg, M., et al., 2010. Left is where the L is right. Significantly delayed reaction time in limb laterality recognition in both CRPS and phantom limb pain patients. *Neuroscience Letters* 486 (3):240–5.

Saragiotto, B. T., Maher, C. G., Yamato, T. P., et al., 2016. Motor control exercise for chronic non-specific low-back pain. *Cochrane Database of Systematic Reviews* (1):CD012004.

Stronks, H. C., Walker, J., Parker, D. J., et al., 2017. Training improves vibrotactile spatial acuity and intensity discrimination on the lower back using coin motors. *Artificial Organs* 41 (11):1059–70.

Wand, B. M., James, M., Abbaszadeh, S., et al., 2014. Assessing self-perception in patients with chronic low back pain: development of a back-specific body-perception questionnaire. *Journal of Back and Musculoskeletal Rehabilitation* 27 (4):463–73.

Wang, Q., Guo, Z. L., Yu, Y. B., et al., 2018. Two-point discrimination predicts pain relief after lower limb nerve decompression for painful diabetic peripheral neuropathy. *Plastic and Reconstructive Surgery* 141 (3):397e–403e.

Wolny, T., Saulicz, E., Linek, P., et al., 2016. Effect of manual therapy and neurodynamic techniques vs ultrasound and laser on 2PD in patients with CTS: A randomized controlled trial. *Journal of Hand Therapy,* 29 (3):235–45.

14
Case Examples

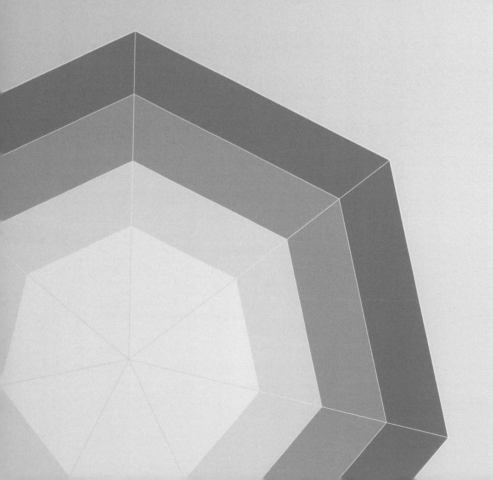

The preceding chapters describe different strategies, tools and observations intended to help clinicians build a phenotype of patients with musculoskeletal pain conditions, with the goal of determining the primary drivers of the individual patient's pain experience. But beyond just building a profile, we have also indicated that many of the same clinical signs and tools can be used to predict some aspects of a patient's future. In this way, the concept of the radar plot and phenotyping can be used for decisions about both intervention and prognosis/theranosis. In the acute stage of injury, we believe the value of the radar plot will be found in its ability to estimate the most likely trajectory a patient is going to follow during their course of recovery, and in those who are expected to follow a more problematic course, can provide the reasons for *why* recovery is unlikely or slow to occur. In the chronic pain state, the question is slightly different – we already know the intermediate-term prognosis was poor, so the natural clinical course (prognosis) is less relevant. In this population, the more valuable contribution is to address the question: How likely is it that this patient will respond to my intervention?

Here we provide two cases: an acute and chronic case whereby the phenotyping process is revealed through active listening, historical information relayed by the patient, findings from clinical tests, and outcomes on screening tools and patient-reported outcome measures. Next, we ask the reader to try triangulating the available information to build their own radar plot of the patient's pain experience whereby a more informed plan of care can be developed. We have attempted to model this after more real-world examples where not all information will be hand-fed. With knowledge of existing evidence, some intuition, and listening for meaning as well as content, we believe you'll be able to create useful radar plots from these cases.

Acute case

Jan is a 34-year-old Caucasian female. Seven days ago, she was the belted driver of a 4-door sedan that was stopped in traffic when impacted from behind on the right side by a sport utility vehicle (SUV) traveling at an estimated 40 km/h (~25 mph). She reports that her headrest was well adjusted, and she was looking forward but was unaware of the impending impact. She denies loss of consciousness. The airbag deployed in the 'bullet' vehicle and there was substantial damage to both vehicles; so much so that both were written off. Both drivers were taken to the emergency medicine department of a large tertiary level 1 trauma center and Jan reported immediate neck discomfort that was corroborated by the physician's exam with neck midline tenderness on palpation.

She is younger (per the established CPR), which would immediately be a positive sign with regards to expected recovery.

We have very little confidence that crash-related parameters influence outcomes.

Based on the information, would imaging be considered as being *usually not appropriate, may be appropriate, or usually appropriate*? (Hint: look at the Canadian C-Spine and Nexus rules online, using the information we just provided.)

Computed tomography (CT) of the head and neck was performed in the emergency department. Findings ruled out significant pathology for fracture, but the radiology report listed multi-level facet joint arthropathy and mild central stenosis.

There were no indications suggesting fracture or ligamentous insufficiency, but how might the reported findings of facet joint arthropathy and mild significant central stenosis frame your discussions with Jan OR potentially her perceptions of her spine health since the crash?

She was discharged with simple analgesics and informed to follow-up with her family physician if symptoms persisted. Symptoms of constant stiffness and intermittent right-sided headaches began the following day and have worsened over the following 48 h motivating her to see her family physician. She received a diagnosis of whiplash associated disorder grade II (mobility deficits and tenderness to palpation but no neurological signs). She was referred to physical therapy for modalities and unsupervised exercise, massage, and received NSAIDs (ibuprofen). Upon presentation to the clinic, Jan reports average neck discomfort as ~4/10, ranging from 2/10 at its best and 5–6/10 at its worst. You ask her to complete the Neck Disability Index (NDI) revealing a score of 23/50 (or 46%). She reports feeling frightened to drive, even as a passenger.

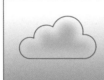

Interpret her pain and NDI ratings in light of the known prognostic information presented earlier in this book (see Fig. 5.2).

Despite the fact she reports being active (goes to Yoga 3 days/week and is the social chair of her son's competitive swim team) she has yet to return to her pre-collision job of traveling regional sales supervisor for an auto parts plant, complaining of ongoing neck pain and headaches as well as sensitivity to light and difficulty concentrating that worsens after a couple hours of work. She is happily married and prior to her injury she contributed equally to the family's finances. She is an excellent historian and informs, in unsolicited fashion, her mother was killed in a car crash 22 years ago involving a large truck that ran a red light. Her father never remarried, raising Jan and her older sister (now 38) by himself. She frequently worries about the same fate for her and her loved ones. She does not take any medications beyond the NSAIDs.

On clinical examination cervical mobility is limited in all planes with no other obvious mechanical pattern. She appears to be tender to palpation anywhere in the neck or shoulder girdle region, even flinching at times in response to light touch over these regions. Her body diagram reveals pain that is situated on both sides of her neck, right temporal and occipital region, right > left shoulder girdle, diffuse right upper arm, and the thoracolumbar region. She reports sleeping 4–5 hours per night since the crash, but also states that even at the best of times, her sleep has never been more than 5 hours per night as she is a 'light sleeper'.

What key features of her experience thus far could inform your assessment?

What self-report measures might you choose to collect beyond those already provided?

You decide to test pressure pain detection threshold, which reveals widespread sensory hypersensitivity (local to the neck and over tibialis anterior). Her pain thresholds decrease (more sensitive) following 3 min of moderately vigorous stationary cycling. Joint position sense error (nominating the center of a target after returning from cervical rotation with the eyes closed) and two-point discrimination are both impaired compared to population norms but near the high ends of normal. She further informs that she has difficulty with reading for pleasure in that her eyes quickly fatigue and this brings on her headache and diffuse pain.

On self-report measures she has: Pain Catastrophizing Scale score of 12/52 (low), a score on the self-report version of the Leeds Assessment of Neuropathic Signs and Symptoms of 6/24 (six points under the cut score of 12/24), and her scores on the Patient Health Questionnaire-9 indicate a potential depressive disorder (right at the threshold for a positive screen, but no suicidal ideation).

She reports generally good relationships with her insurer, her husband, co-workers, and family doctor. However, she indicates her son is very worried about her and her health. Jan then describes feeling pressured and scrutinized by her employer to return to work. She reports experiencing increasing financial hardship due to medical/rehabilitation expenses and lost wages.

Use the information you've gleaned from Jan's case to create your own radar plot – a blank triangulation table and radar plot are provided in Box 14.1.

Highlight those drivers in which you've got enough information to triangulate your findings, indicating confidence in your level for that domain. Note that it is possible to be confident that a certain domain is not a primary driver if enough evidence to the contrary is present. After you've completed this, turn to p. 189 for an example table and plot that we've created for this case.

Box 14.1 Exercise: Jan's radar plot

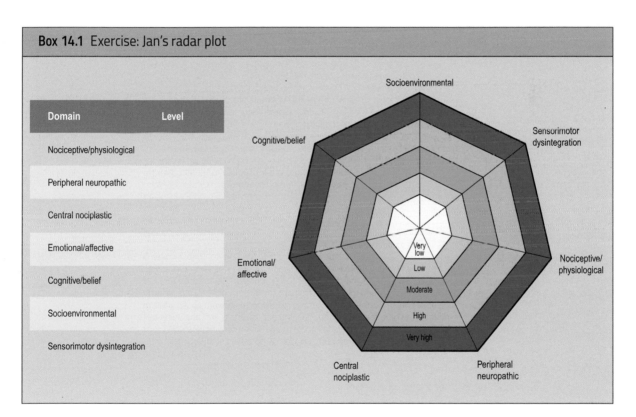

Domain	Level
Nociceptive/physiological	
Peripheral neuropathic	
Central nociplastic	
Emotional/affective	
Cognitive/belief	
Socioenvironmental	
Sensorimotor dysintegration	

Chronic case

Mohan, a 45-year-old chartered professional accountant, presents to your practice seeking more information and recommendations to address his long 5-year history of bilateral low back and buttock pain. He has sought and received care from several prior healthcare providers from a variety of disciplines, including a physical therapist, chiropractor, massage therapist, acupuncturist, and osteopath with most providing at best short-term relief. After having a consultation with a spine surgeon 2½ years ago who indicated he was not a good candidate for surgery as he was deemed 'not impaired enough', he has been managed primarily by his family doctor through NSAIDs and low-dose opioids to maintain his daily function and allow him to continue to work and earn an income. He reports doing his best to remain active and enjoys going for walks in the evening with his wife and dog, though often requires his wife to hold the dog's leash.

His goals for visiting you today are to seek your opinions on what may be causing his pain, get some advice and recommendations for additional management strategies, and wants to know whether you expect his condition can improve. When pressed, improvement in his mind would be less frequent pain that, when it does occur, is less intense and does not interfere with his daily activities. He'd like to be able to sleep more comfortably, and to take up a more active lifestyle. He has enjoyed cycling in the past and would like to get back to doing so at or around the level he did in his mid-30s.

Duration 5 years: While this doesn't rule out a nociceptive driver, it makes the likelihood of a central nociplastic or sensorimotor dysintegration driver more likely.

Age 45 years: It would be reasonable to expect some positive imaging findings on x-ray, CT, or MRI, though in the absence of a clear association between a structural pathology and some aspect of his clinical presentation, we should also expect that in isolation such findings may be incidental and may not be relevant to your plan of care. However, imaging findings may still be important especially as multiple cumulative findings appear to increase the risk of recurrence of low back pain in the future.

Chartered professional accountant: Mohan will have a post-secondary education and would likely be classed somewhere in between a middle- and upper-class socioeconomic status. These tend to be good prognostic/theranostic indicators. The fact that he continues to work is, by definition, a good prognostic indicator for work status in the future.

He verbally reports and visually details on a body diagram that his pain is in the bilateral low back and buttock regions. He informs that he manages his pain and function adequately well with NSAIDs and opioids.

Pain location: Hard to place this right now, though the description of the pain in a fairly localized region is at least *not* strongly indicative of widespread sensory hypersensitivity.

Pharmaceuticals: Plenty to think about here. Are the NSAIDs effective? If so, this would point more towards a peripheral nociceptive pain driver. Are they ineffective? Is it the opioids that are having the effect? Are either having an effect? Has anyone checked the medications recently or tried to taper one or the other? More information is needed than we can glean from this initial consultation, but it certainly provides an area for further exploration.

An interesting side note arises here in that he feels as though he needs his wife to hold the dog leash. Why does he feel as though he cannot/should not hold the leash? Fear of pain is something that we'd start to think about, though we'll need more information to know if it's a rational or irrational fear. Another question might be what effect does walking have on his pain? If it relieves the pain, this may point us in the direction of a more nociceptive driver. If not, perhaps more central.

He is married: We perhaps need not dive too deeply here, but simple questions such as 'Is your wife healthy? Is she able to help out around the home?' may bring to light information regarding the nature of the relationship, and perhaps other health conditions that Mohan is faced with daily. An additional question would be whether he has any children and whether they are supportive.

Mohan details his feelings about healthcare professionals in that he often views them as 'the experts' and that he puts a lot of emphasis on the information he receives from them, as well as doing a lot of research on 'low back pain' on the internet. (Knowing what kinds of information he has received from these prior providers could help us to understand the cognitive drivers of his pain experience.)

Past medical history, general health status, and observations

Mohan states that his pain started five years ago and while he's not entirely sure of the cause, he knows it was two days after he helped a friend move house. His initial diagnosis from the family doctor was that he *likely over-strained the back muscles* and at the time he was prescribed some NSAIDs and muscle relaxants. Despite expectations that it would be short-lived, the pain did not subside and two weeks later he had his wife drive him to the local emergency department (ED) after he ended up 'flat on my back and couldn't move' in the middle of tying his shoes. He received an MRI while in the ED that revealed 'bulging' intervertebral discs at several levels of his lumbar spine, some degeneration, and something referred to as 'facet arthropathy' (which he has since spent a fair bit of time exploring online). The ED physicians provided him a prescription for a week's worth of long-acting oxycodone and turned his care back to his family doctor who has maintained his pharmaceutical management ever since. He states that the combination of NSAIDs and oxycodone took the edge off the pain such that he was able to return to work four days later and has not missed a day since.

Onset: The mechanism of onset here is somewhat unclear, though he seems to be linking it to a delayed reaction from an intensive day of lifting and carrying while helping a friend move.

While not diagnostic, a strong nociceptive driver might be more likely if he were to state that his pain started immediately during a discrete event (e.g. an awkward lift and twist).

Meaning and understanding: We'd be slightly concerned about the messaging offered, or at least how it had been interpreted, from his prior encounters with general and emergency physicians. Exploring his illness representations (how he makes sense of his pain) seems like a priority focus.

Ongoing management: While it's nice to know he has a strategy that he can use for relief of his pain, we would like to see him armed with other options for those times when the medications are either not enough, or in the case that he is interested in trying to taper. His interest in walking and cycling may be directions to keep in mind.

He states that his pain is usually worse in the morning when getting out of bed, fluctuates slightly over the course of the day, and worsens again later in the day, and this is fairly consistent. He denies numbness or paresthesia in his extremities. He states he is currently able to do most of the things he needs to do in an average day but does so 'carefully and slowly'. He rates his current pain at an intensity of 5 on a 0–10 Numeric Rating Scale and indicates that over the past 48 hours it has fluctuated from 0/10 (he can sometimes forget about it when he's 'in a flow' at work) to 8/10, especially in the mornings. He states he experiences pain about 60% of the time on a usual day.

Mohan reports being otherwise healthy, though he takes atorvastatin (Lipitor) for slightly elevated blood cholesterol. At 5 feet 10 inches tall and weighing 206 pounds (178 cm and 93.5kg) his BMI places him about 30–35 lbs (13.5–16kg) overweight and he is aware that he has gained weight since his pain started. He states his cardiovascular system is otherwise healthy having recently had a physical examination. His diet is a mixture of foods from his native India and those of his adopted North American homeland.

On observation you note that he tends to move in a somewhat slow and guarded fashion though is generally willing to perform the movements you ask of him during your clinical assessment. He tends to use his hands to support himself as he bends over and straightens back up, and you see him wincing from time to time during movement.

Pain behavior: while pain ratings are notoriously difficult to interpret, the fact that he is able to describe a consistent daily pattern of fluctuation, and that it fits with what would make biological sense for a nociceptive (inflammatory in this case) driver, provides support for that type of driver.

The other pain indicators, including intensity and frequency, given that his pain is chronic, provide little direction for phenotyping. However, they offer potentially useful measures for evaluating the effectiveness of your intervention, especially if you can capture these in an adequately valid and reliable way.

Weight: We're not going to put undue emphasis on this and there is no need to shame someone where it's not due. The evidence to suggest that weight loss will lead to reduced back pain, especially in someone who is only modestly overweight, is weak at best. This is little more than a secondary consideration at this stage.

Nutrition: In the future we may have more information to guide our decisions regarding nutrition and back pain, but at this time we'll simply recognize that he appears to have a reasonably varied diet, at least as much as most North Americans do.

Movement analysis: The slow guarded movements could point us in several directions. Is there a discrete, consistent, and biomechanically meaningful pattern to his pain with movement? If so, a nociceptive driver may be indicated. Could this represent fear of pain (cognitive driver)? A self-report tool or asking him about his symptoms may shed more light here. Could this be a learned coping behavior over time, that allows him to do the things he wants to do if perhaps a bit more slowly and uncomfortably than normal (cognitive or emotional driver)? Is this something someone else told him to do (socioenvironmental driver)? More information is needed here.

From this example we hope to illustrate how considerable information can be gleaned from even routine questioning and simple movement observations. There are several pieces of information here, most of which seem to indicate a primary nociceptive driver, though there are some that might indicate otherwise, and the duration of the symptoms would suggest this is not a *purely* nociceptive driver. This is the value of using multiple information sources (that need not be burdensome) and of grading your confidence in each driver on some kind of graduated scale, like the radar plot does. Here, you may not be confident in a 'very high' nociceptive driver (especially given the chronicity), though you may be confident in a moderate or even high driver, and a low or moderate central nociplastic driver. Other tests and questions will continue to hone your clinical impression as get you closer to the most optimal drivers to address first. Your intervention decisions should then naturally flow from there.

Use the information you've gleaned from Mohan's case to create your own radar plot – a blank triangulation table and radar plot are provided in Box 14.2. Highlight those drivers in which you've got enough information to triangulate your findings, indicating confidence in your level for that domain. Note that it is possible to be confident that a certain domain is not a primary driver if enough evidence to the contrary is present. After you've completed this, turn to p. 189 for an example table and plot that we've created for this case.

Box 14.2 Exercise: Mohan's radar plot

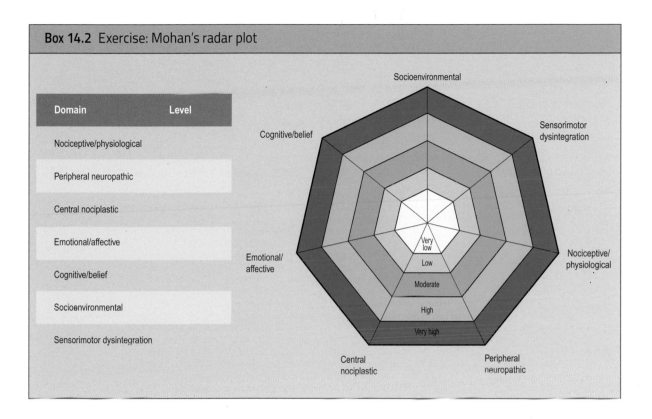

Domain	Level
Nociceptive/physiological	
Peripheral neuropathic	
Central nociplastic	
Emotional/affective	
Cognitive/belief	
Socioenvironmental	
Sensorimotor dysintegration	

Concluding remarks

You'll likely notice that there is some ambiguity around creating your radar plot for these cases, just as there will be for your patients. This is both intentional and necessary, as the field of pain management is also very ambiguous despite ongoing attempts to reduce it to individual components. To become comfortable helping people to manage their pain you must yourself become comfortable with uncertainty. Remember McCaffery: *pain is what the patient says it is, and occurs when he or she says it does* (McCaffery, 1968). You may start asking yourself questions like: how can scores on maladaptive cognition tools be low but scores on emotional screening tools be high? How should I consider the effect of cognitions in the presence of strong socioenvironmental drivers? Are central nociplastic drivers not just a subtype of sensorimotor dysintegration?

We hope you are asking these questions, as it suggests you are thinking critically about the nature of pain assessment, prognosis, and treatment. Even the very nature of our existing knowledge around much of what we think of as pain is open to questioning and debate. Is there even such a thing as causation in pain, assuming we could find it if there was? These are questions for which philosophers and social scientists need to engage with basic and clinical scientists to explore, trouble, and challenge all of the pre-existing assumptions about what is pain and what is knowledge about pain. We hope that by the next iteration of this book this type of engagement will have become the norm, though we currently hold only mild optimism that it will occur.

The radar plot is not a panacea. It is meant to provide a framework for clinicians attempting to make at least *some* sense out of a highly complex field of human experience. It is a step in the right direction, but it is not the final solution. We believe that if clinicians can begin thinking in the terms presented here, and start capturing clinical data routinely, then the radar plot can be better conceptualized as a bridge between the *old ways* of placing all patients into a few discrete subcategories, and what will inevitably become a new practice of augmented rehabilitation through use of advanced artificial intelligence. The concept of phenotyping feels to us like a lovely evolution of current practice towards what we anticipate will be even more advances in the next 10–20 years. We hope you find the same, and ultimately, we hope that with the radar plot you and your patients are better able to work together as partners in effective pain assessment, prediction, and treatment.

Reference

McCaffery, M.,1968. Nursing practice theories related to cognition, bodily pain, and man- environment interactions. Los Angeles: University of California at Los Angeles Students' Store.

Box 14.3 Jan's completed table and radar plot

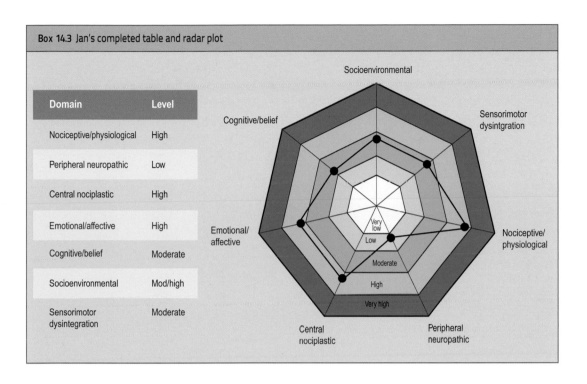

Domain	Level
Nociceptive/physiological	High
Peripheral neuropathic	Low
Central nociplastic	High
Emotional/affective	High
Cognitive/belief	Moderate
Socioenvironmental	Mod/high
Sensorimotor dysintegration	Moderate

Box 14.4 Mohan's completed table and radar plot

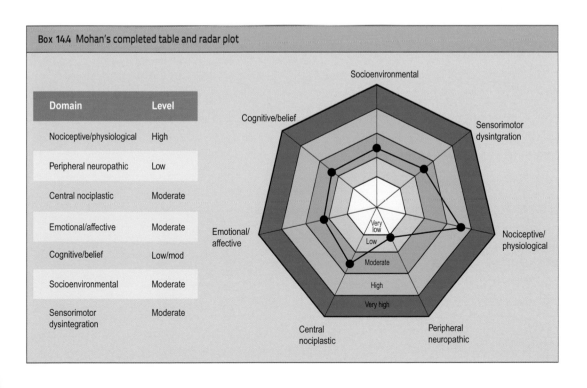

Domain	Level
Nociceptive/physiological	High
Peripheral neuropathic	Low
Central nociplastic	Moderate
Emotional/affective	Moderate
Cognitive/belief	Low/mod
Socioenvironmental	Moderate
Sensorimotor dysintegration	Moderate

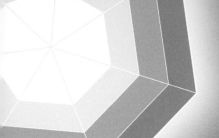

Note: page numbers followed by b, f, or t indicate a box, figure, or table, respectively

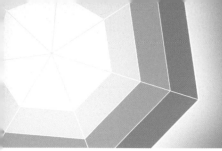